JANIS POWERS

HEALTH CARE

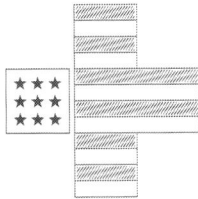

MEET THE

AMERICAN

DREAM

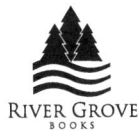

RIVER GROVE
BOOKS

Published by River Grove Books
Austin, TX
www.rivergrovebooks.com

Distributed by River Grove Books

Design and composition by Greenleaf Book Group
Cover design by Greenleaf Book Group
Figures and charts ©Janis Powers

Publisher's Cataloging-in-Publication data is available.

Print ISBN: 978-1-63299-195-9

eBook ISBN: 978-1-63299-196-6

First Edition

Health Care: Meet the American Dream is dedicated to those who challenge the status quo with rigorous, fact-based debate and an open mind. Challenging the status quo doesn't mean we simply critique it. It's our responsibility to come up with creative solutions to improve it.

"If everybody is thinking alike, then somebody isn't thinking."

—GENERAL GEORGE S. PATTON JR.

CONTENTS

PREFACE ix

ACKNOWLEDGMENTS xv

PART 1   **America's Health Care System: Today**

INTRO   The ER: A Case Study in Misaligned Incentives 3

CH 1   Health Care Primer: Understanding Health
Care's Unique Language 15

CH 2   The Money: Where It All Goes 31

CH 3   A Historical View of Health Policy:
How Did Things Get So Complicated? 45

CH 4   Perspectives on Health Insurance 55

CH 5   Attempts at Health Care Transformation 65

CH 6   The Case Against a Single Payer System 71

CH 7   Value-Based Care: An Academic Policy Solution 79

PART 2   **America's Health Care System: The Dream Plan**

INTRO   A Blue Sky Proposal 87

CH 8   Longitudinal Health Care Plan 91

CH 9   The Obsolescence of Traditional Health Insurance 109

CH 10   Business Case for the LHCP 129

CH 11   How the Dream Plan Can Reduce
Costs in Health Care 139

CH 12   Public Health 153

CH 13   Making or Breaking: Critical Success Factors 163

CH 14   Recommendations for Short-Term Change 175

CONCLUSION 183

NOTES 185

LHCP BUSINESS CASE DETAIL 201

ABOUT THE AUTHOR 207

PREFACE

I have spent my career as a health care consultant specializing in strategy and operations. In layman's terms, I advise hospitals, ambulatory surgery centers, and other providers about how market pressures, new technology, and policy changes will impact their business. My goal is to help my clients use their financial resources to provide the best care to as many patients in the most effective manner possible. I am an efficiency expert with a heart. Every dollar wasted in the health care system is a dollar that could be spent improving the life of someone else.

Over the course of my career, I've worked for clients all over the United States, including the nation's largest for-profit and not-for-profit systems. I've consulted for academic medical centers ("teaching hospitals") in the urban core and federally qualified health clinics in rural America. I've analyzed every major department in a hospital. I can look at a floor plan of an ambulatory surgery center and tell you if it's going to make money or lose it. This deep, hands-on expertise enables me to understand the day-to-day impact that new laws and policies will have on all constituents in the health care system—patients, providers, government, employers, insurance companies, and pharmaceutical companies.

Despite this experience, I have never been an employee of a hospital, an insurance company, or any government organization. Aside from a short stint as a director of business development for a health care start-up, I have spent my career as a consultant to, not an employee of, the health care industry. I bring a perspective that is not clouded by training or loyalty to any aspect of the health care establishment.

Further, I don't have any degrees in medicine, public health, public policy, or social work. In college I majored in architecture at Yale and have masters' degrees in architecture and business from the University of Michigan. My academic training relates to how different aspects of a system must collaborate to create a harmonious whole. I think about how things work, how much they cost, how people are impacted by their surroundings, and what drives human behavior. I've been perfectly trained to study the health care industry despite the fact that I had no intention of doing it when I was enrolled in school.

I am a proud American, and my appreciation for our country has been solidified by decades of travel around the world. I have been to over thirty-five countries. My first trip outside the United States was a family "vacation" to the Union of Soviet Socialist Republics in 1977 during the height of the Cold War. I was seven years old. I learned that there are human beings behind politics, people behave like their neighbors, and history and geography define the culture of a people. These are all the feature functions that impact health care—no matter where in the world you happen to be.

This book is the culmination of years of thinking about ways to fix the American health care system with a solution that is truly American. I believe that a health care system that satisfies the needs of Americans must be based on our distinct social doctrine. My concept, called the Dream Plan, uses the precepts of the American Dream—individuality, self-determination, and community support—as inspiration for a new model of health care.

■ ■ ■

The American Dream is the hallowed ideology that any individual can advance his or her state of being through ambition and hard work. It defines the American psyche. Historian James Truslow Adams used the phrase in his 1931 book *The Epic of America* in which he wrote,

"The American Dream is that dream of a land in which life should be better and richer and fuller for everyone, with opportunity for each according to ability or achievement."

Achieving success through personal industry is a source of pride in our country. We love stories of self-made men and women, people who have empowered themselves to reach their goals. It is one of the few concepts that is truly bipartisan. Virtually all politicians can bolster voter enthusiasm simply by mentioning the phrase.

It is also one of the few ideologies that transcends gender, race, income, religious affiliation, sexual orientation, or virtually any mechanism for population segmentation. Each of us has our own interpretation of the American Dream. It is informed by our personal experiences and unique to each of us. Some of us may hope to buy a home, others to send a child to college, start a business, or become a millionaire. The common thread is that we believe we have the power to positively impact our future through a self-determined level of commitment.

The Dream Plan gives each of us an eye into our future with information that empowers us to be in charge of our destiny—how we want to interact with the health care system, how we want to spend our resources, and how we want to live and die. The plan charges us to work in concert with the medical professionals who can guide us to make the best decisions. We'll need the government to provide restrained oversight related to consumer protections, safety, and ensuring fair access to care. But accountability for health outcomes lies with the American people. Each of us must be motivated to be as healthy as we can be.

. . .

The Dream Plan puts forth an alternative to the health care system we have today. Private health insurance, Medicare, and Medicaid would no longer exist. Instead of paying third parties—insurance companies and the government—to pay providers for our care, we'd pay the providers directly. The Dream Plan removes the "middle man" from the equation by creating a system that allows Americans to save all the money they'll need to pay for their health care over the course of their lives. Those who cannot save the resources required, or who are afflicted with serious medical conditions, will be covered in a public health program. The Dream Plan ensures that all Americans will be accounted for in the health care system. No one gets left behind.

The Dream Plan outlines the parameters for a new type of product called a Longitudinal Health Care Plan, or LHCP. Americans will access LHCPs similar to how they would enroll in an insurance plan or set up a bank account. LHCP providers (who may wind up being insurers and banks) would offer these products to customers to help them manage their money so they can manage their health.

LHCPs will replace traditional health insurance because health insurance will soon be obsolete. Advancements in genetic testing and predictive analytics will enable each of us to learn which diseases we're predisposed to develop and when. The Dream Plan takes this technology and puts it on steroids, providing LHCP customers with a detailed understanding of their future health care conditions. Once people are empowered with this information, they won't need comprehensive insurance. The money that individuals previously paid to an insurer and some of what goes to the government will now go into an LHCP to be invested for their own future health care needs.

The Dream Plan addresses two major imperatives for change: the general unhealthiness of the American populace and our inefficient, financially misaligned health care system. We cannot look to the successful models of care that have been deployed in other countries and apply them at home, because no other country in the world is like America. Rather, in order to fix the health care system, we must reaffirm our American values. The principles that define the American spirit should also define how the American health care system works and how we, as citizens, relate to it.

As Americans, we have a responsibility to live healthy lives and to contribute to a positive and productive society. We must take more accountability for our individual health by focusing on prevention and wellness. It is imperative that we also support each other in our quest to elevate the greater good. Our health care system needs to be structured in a way that promotes these values so we can redirect the excessive amounts we spend on treating our sickness to investing in our people, education, infrastructure, innovation, and safety.

Health care: Meet the American Dream.

ACKNOWLEDGMENTS

I would like to acknowledge the support, patience, and kindness of my family, friends, and colleagues. You all know that I say what I mean. Much of what I've said is now in a book. Let the debate begin!

Special thanks to—

My children, Veronica and Barrett, for allowing me to explain the seemingly endless string of editorials that I cut from the newspaper and hang on the refrigerator. May your horizons continue to expand as you explore the world.

Stephanie and Jeff Mims for treating me like family.

Cynthia Kinnas for encouraging me to try new things.

Dr. David Feldman. May we always break bread together.

PART ONE

AMERICA'S
HEALTH CARE SYSTEM

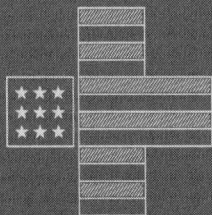

TODAY

THE ER: A CASE STUDY IN MISALIGNED INCENTIVES

Miracles are performed every day in emergency rooms (ERs). Fast-acting, amazing medical professionals resuscitate, diagnose, and treat patients who have arrived in ERs—some of them on the verge of death. Highly trained staff combine encyclopedic clinical knowledge with cutting-edge technology and techniques—and they save lives. We've all seen the shows, from the genre-defining hit *ER* to the recent series *Code Black*. The ER—as portrayed for and perceived by the masses—presents health care in America at its best.

But when health care strategists like myself evaluate ERs, we view them as emblematic of so much that is wrong with our health care system. I'm not talking about the quality of care delivered at the point of service. ER physicians, nurses, and staff are, for the most part, some of the most devoted and talented practitioners in the system. I'm referring to the financial and behavioral ecosystem that surrounds the delivery of care in the ER. It's a mess.

Emergency rooms are designed to respond to unexpected life-and-death situations. Staff in the ER never knows what kind of case is going to come through the door at any given moment, so they have to be prepared for everything. They need 24/7 access to advanced diagnostic equipment, fully equipped operating rooms, a comprehensive spectrum of medications, any number of specialty supplies, and of course—physicians and staff trained to provide the emergency care. This is why the ER is the costliest place in the health care system to deliver care.

What goes on in and around the emergency room is a case study in how each of health care's major constituents behave in ways contrary to their professional and personal missions. Hospitals, insurers, the government, physicians, and patients each engage in activities that sacrifice care quality and/or drive up costs. I've highlighted some of the issues that are regularly identified as problems as a means to provide some insights into the complexity of the health care system.

CASE #1: WELL-INTENTIONED, FINANCIALLY ONEROUS LEGISLATION

The major problem in the ER setting is that people with gunshot wounds and victims of heart attacks aren't the only ones who show up. Patients come if they think they've sprained their ankle, or they spike a fever, or have a headache. High-cost venues like emergency rooms should be the site of last resort for these types of nonemergency health care issues.

The root cause of this situation is the Emergency Medical Treatment and Labor Act (EMTALA)[1] that was enacted in 1986. The law requires any hospital that accepts Medicare reimbursement (and the vast majority of them do) to treat any patient with an identifiable emergency condition who arrives at the hospital's ER. Medical care must be provided to that patient, regardless of the patient's ability to pay.

The intent of the law was to make sure that the health care system didn't shut people out and that access to health care would be provided to anyone. To those in America who clamor for "universal health care," please take note. We already have it. It's called the emergency room.

While ensuring access to care is a good thing, figuring out how to pay for it is one of our nation's most significant challenges. EMTALA's solution was to make hospitals pay for it—with some help. Just prior to the time that EMTALA was passed, the government had developed a way for hospitals to be compensated for the high volume of care they were delivering to Medicaid and uninsured patients. Criteria were developed to pay hospitals Disproportionate Share Hospital (DSH, pronounced "dish") payments for this care. Over the decades, hospitals have become increasingly reliant on DSH payments as an important source of revenue.

In 2010, the Affordable Care Act was passed, and it altered the expectation that hospitals would need DSH payments. ACA's intent—similar to that of EMTALA—was to ensure that all Americans would have access to health care. The ACA used several strategies to bring "universal health care" coverage to America. In particular, the ACA called for the voluntary expansion of the Medicaid program to cover selected low-income, uninsured Americans. It also included the *individual mandate*, which required every American to purchase health insurance or face a financial penalty.

Put yourself in the mind of an ACA policy designer in, say, 2008. You're creating a system that you hope will lead to universal health care coverage. In that scenario, everyone would have some sort of health insurance. Therefore, there would be no need to compensate hospitals for the charity care they deliver, so hospitals wouldn't need DSH payments. So, as part of ACA, the amount of DSH payments passed on to most hospitals was supposed to be cut.

ACA's goals were noble, but as of the first quarter of 2018, almost 16%[2] of non-elderly adults (meaning those who do not qualify for Medicare) still didn't have health insurance. Aware of the situation, the government has postponed the planned reductions to DSH payments several times. Yet the threat of the cuts looms large as pressure is mounting to put more controls on health care spending.

These regulatory issues put hospitals in a real ethical and financial bind when it comes to treating nonemergency and nonpaying patients in an ER. Doctors are bound by the Hippocratic Oath, which commits them to ensuring the safety and well-being of patients. The mission of most hospitals around the world is to provide care for patients with dignity and compassion. Care comes first; payment comes second.

CASE #2: PRICE LISTS WITH INFLATED, NONSENSICAL PRICING

But hospitals are finding ways to make sure they get paid. And their strategies to do so are far from virtuous.

Hospitals use a complicated set of factors to develop their own unique pricing structures. These prices are listed on what's called the hospital's *charge master*. Charge masters are not universally reviewed by third-party industry groups or regulated by the federal government. The main use of the charge master is to serve as a starting point for negotiations with payers (insurance companies) for the rates hospitals will be paid for care. Payers often opt to pay a percentage off the charge master, meaning that a hospital will get paid, say, 70% of the "list price" for a procedure or group of services. Therefore, the rates on the charge master are set very high because hospitals know they'll get pushed down in negotiations.

But patients don't know this. They may get a bill that has charge master-based pricing on it. An uninsured patient may be on the hook for the entire bill, which could run into tens of thousands of dollars.

Even people who are insured rarely have 100% of their emergency room charges covered, especially if they don't end up being admitted to the hospital. This means that even those people who have paid for insurance coverage usually have to pay a percentage of the charges they rack up—this can often equal 20, 30, or even 50% of the bill for their emergency room care. Depending on the situation, the bill may be reflective of charges based on the insurer's negotiated rates with the hospital, the charge master rates, or something in between.

Most patients don't realize that they can negotiate these charges. And even if they did, many lack the sophistication and wherewithal to do it. Patients would have to appeal their case to the hospital's administration. They'll have the most luck if they can demonstrate that they are in financial distress and cannot cover the bill. At this point, the hospital might lower the rates it will charge the patient based on another independently determined price structure called a *sliding fee scale*. At a high level, this price list tries to match a patient's income level with the charges the hospital thinks the patient should pay.

Patients can protest the rates on other grounds, like comparing the rates they've been charged to those of other providers in the market, but all of these negotiations take time and fortitude, and not all patients are successful. This is one of the reasons that charges for emergency room services were considered the number one reason why individuals have trouble paying for their medical bills.[3]

CASE #3: PROVIDERS WITH DIFFERENT CONTRACTS SERVING THE SAME PATIENT

One of the most maddening ER billing situations is the doctor/hospital contracting conflict called *balance billing*. This is a scenario where the patient's insurer has a contract with the hospital for emergency services, but it doesn't have one with the physician in the ER who winds up treating the patient. In such cases, the doctor is considered "out of network." The patient will receive a separate bill for the doctor's services. Oftentimes, the physician will bill at an exorbitant rate—similar to the charge master pricing used by hospitals.

In other words, the hospital may have a contract with an insurer like Aetna. Aetna may also offer a contract to a physician so patients can use his or her services. But if the physician doesn't like the terms of the Aetna deal, he or she is under no obligation to agree to it. However, the hospital may nonetheless grant the physician the privileges to work at the hospital. This creates an element of confusion that only adds to an already stressful situation for patients and their families.

Balance billing is a hot topic in many legislative communities.[4] It is a situation that is difficult to resolve because both the hospital and the physician contract with payers independently. The hospital cannot require the physician to enter into a contractual agreement with the payers of the hospital's choosing and vice versa.

CASE #4: SELLING CONVENIENCE BUT IGNORING ITS COST

Hospitals are motivated to maximize the number of patients who go through their emergency rooms so they can cover the high fixed costs associated with treatment. Think of an ER like a manufacturing plant. The per-unit cost of making a widget goes down as more and more widgets are made. That's because the high fixed cost of the plant can be allocated to the large number of widgets in production. The same is true for the ER. In high-level terms, the more patients the ER treats, the lower the per-patient cost of care delivery will be for the facility.

Many hospitals turn to advertising to drive volume (pun intended) into their emergency rooms. Perhaps you've seen magazine ads, billboards, or social media posts promoting the convenience of a local hospital's ER. Some electronic ads note the current wait times at their facilities. These billboards aren't posted to help ambulance drivers figure out which hospital can treat their flatlining passenger the quickest. These ads are designed to draw nonemergent cases into the ER.

And it works—because it's convenient to patients and to their caregivers. Consider this scenario. It's six o'clock in the evening, and a working parent's child has a fever and a phlegmy cough. If the child is sick the next day, the parent has to stay home from work, losing a day's worth of pay. The sooner the child can be diagnosed, the quicker the child can start treatment. That speeds up the child's recovery time, which reduces the parent's time away from work. That parent wants that child treated ASAP.

A parent may compare a typical ER co-pay of $100 to a day's wages and opt for the ER visit. Yes, there's the potential for a big fat bill on the back end, but people are more motivated by convenience and immediacy. And since most folks don't clearly understand the coverage provided by their insurance company, they'll focus on the short-term health problem, not the longer-term financial one.

CASE #5: THROWING TECHNOLOGY AT THE PROBLEM

Insurers don't want to pay ER rates for nonemergent care that could be delivered in a cheaper, clinic-based environment. For years, insurers have tried to keep these cases out of the ER through a variety of strategies. Patient education about alternatives to the ER is common. Insurers encourage patients to consult with their primary care doctors before heading to the emergency room, and most physician practices have doctors on call 24/7, enabling a patient to talk to a medical professional at any time of the day or night.

A more recent option is the use of telemedicine services, enabling a patient to video chat with a provider. Such person-to-person conversations can help assuage a patient's concerns about what's going on medically with themselves or a loved one. Sometimes a preliminary diagnosis can be made. Even better, a patient may get an appointment scheduled with their primary care doctor during the video consultation.

Insurers like telemedicine because the cost of paying for both a video consult and a clinic-based visit is typically less than a charge for a patient visit to an ER. But some data is indicating that telemedicine actually drives up costs in the system.[5] Telemedicine is convenient, so patients use it, but if the video consult requires the patient to wait until the next day to see a doctor, they oftentimes still go to the ER. Then the insurer winds up paying for the expensive ER visit *and* the telemedicine consult.

CASE #6: PENALIZING PATIENTS FOR NOT BEING DOCTORS

Some insurers aren't waiting to see if telemedicine services can keep nonemergent patients out of the ER. They're simply changing their reimbursement practices with the intent of changing patient behavior. Over the past few years, some insurers have begun to institute policies that penalize patients for inappropriate ER usage. A number of plans affiliated with the Blue Cross Blue Shield Association feel so strongly about patient abuse of the emergency room that they have instituted policies denying payments for ER visits that they deem to be unnecessary.[6]

Insurers have provided data to show what they consider to be out-of-control ER service abuse. A Blue Cross Blue Shield study of New York State emergency rooms from 2013 determined that 90% of the emergency room visits were potentially avoidable.[7] Their interpretation of such a study led them to declare that they'd overpaid for the care for the 90% of patients who could have been treated outside of the ER. The problem with this sort of analysis is that it's retrospective. The study reviewed the cases *after* they were diagnosed. Since patients aren't doctors, they don't know whether their health issue is critical or not. A headache could just be a headache. Or it could be a brain tumor.

An alternative study took the perspective of the patient. The analysis reviewed patient symptoms prior to diagnosis and determined that 92.5% of cases in the ER were identified as urgent at triage.[8] In other words, almost all the patients who showed up in the ER had symptoms that could have been associated with emergency conditions. Such results imply that the vast majority of patients *should* have shown up in the emergency room.

If two studies indicate conflicting information about what cases are truly urgent, how is a patient supposed to know? Yet insurers are penalizing patients anyway as a means to reduce their payments to hospitals. Such behavior threatens access and reduces the overall quality of care, because patients may avoid getting treatment over concerns about costs or coverage.

CASE #7: SOCIETY'S INABILITY TO MANAGE DEATH

No one likes death. Hospital administrators see every death as a blemish on their clinical performance. Hospitals face financial penalties, oftentimes in the form of reduced payments from Medicare, for poor quality ratings, which can include things like high infection rates, readmitting certain patients within thirty days of discharge from the hospital, and mortality (death) rates. Nursing homes and rehab facilities don't want a death on their books either, so they oftentimes transfer at-risk patients back to hospitals or to other facilities. Heavy regulation contributes to a loss of provider focus on the patient, even though the regulations are supposed to improve patient outcomes.[9]

Many doctors view death as a sign of failure especially when they're practicing in an environment with access to the cutting-edge procedures, technology, and medications that can keep patients alive. In the ER, doctors have fairly free rein to order tests, administer drugs, and engage in life-saving procedures for patients in life-threatening situations (assuming the patient doesn't have a do not resuscitate [DNR] order, which prohibits a medical professional from performing the aforementioned life-saving procedures when the patient's heart has stopped beating or they've stopped breathing).

We all get it when the patient is a nineteen-year-old athlete fighting for his life after being hit by a drunk driver. That young man's life is no less important than that of a ninety-two-year-old patient with dementia and three chronic diseases who arrives in the ER in cardiac arrest. Doctors will try mightily to save her too.

Families do a poor job of handling end-of-life transitions because they don't want or don't know how to make life-or-death decisions for a loved one. They stall, sometimes the patient loses his or her cognitive ability, and in a worst-case scenario, the fate of this cherished shadow of a former mother or father winds up in the hands of a physician with a so-called "God Complex," hell-bent on using every medical means necessary to keep the patient alive. Doctors, patients, and their families must have more frank conversations about how to manage the process of dying. If we approach death with emotional clarity and previously agreed-upon, scenario-based action steps, we will ensure that our loved ones are afforded the dignity they deserve.

This is not what health care in America is supposed to be.

THERE'S A FIX, BUT EVERYONE WOULD HAVE TO AGREE

The problems with the ER are fixable. The key is to recognize that nothing has been able to divert nonemergent cases from showing up in the ER. Not education, not telemedicine, not payment penalties. Americans demand convenience. Rather than fight this reality, insurers and policy makers need to acknowledge and manage it.

The solution is simple, and it's been talked about for decades. We need to implement a "fast-track" in the ER: Diagnose patients when they arrive on-site; divert nonemergent cases to a lower-cost clinic environment that's located either adjacent to the ER or off-site; treat everyone else in the ER.

Unfortunately, implementing such a practical solution has been elusive because it would require all the constituents to work collaboratively to change some aspect of their respective businesses. The situation is exacerbated because, as is typical in health care, care delivery is hyper-local, but administrative decisions are centralized at regional, state, and federal levels. Here are just a few of the things that would have to happen to bring this solution to bear:

1. The federal government would have to repeal or amend EMTALA. That would require a review and potential redefinition of cases that are deemed truly emergent and must be treated in an emergency room setting, and those that are not and could be diverted. Such a discussion would require input from various medical groups, such as the American Medical Association, the American Academy of Emergency Medicine, and the American College of Emergency Physicians, as well as the Department of Health and Human Services, civic organizations, and patient advocacy groups.

2. Hospitals would have to rightsize their ERs. Hospitals would need to conduct an analysis of their emergency room volume to try to determine how big their ERs would need to be to serve only the demand for emergency cases. They would also have to

articulate the volume and type of nonemergency cases that could be diverted elsewhere.

3. Alternative care sites would have to be identified for the diverted, nonemergency cases. Hospitals with a significant volume of cases may wish to develop a well-equipped clinic adjacent to their ERs. Such a proposal would require capital investment for the facility project, as well as costs to address any impacts to licensing or other regulatory requirements. All constituents would have to financially contribute to these projects, as the financial burden should not fall solely on the hospitals.

   Alternatively, cases could be diverted to existing clinics in the community. An analysis of regional clinic capacity would likely need to be conducted to ensure that patients could access care at enough sites at the appropriate operating hours to address their health care needs.

4. Insurers—all of them, including Medicare, Medicaid, and private insurers—would have to develop a tiered pricing structure for emergency care. Rates for reimbursement for care delivered in the emergency room may increase if the patients in the ER should become much more acutely ill and more expensive to care for. A separate rate would need to be defined for those who are triaged but receive their care in an alternative location. Finally, there may be a new rate associated with simply conducting the exam to triage the patient. These classifications should be established on an industry-wide basis to simplify payments between providers and insurers.

5. A national patient education program would have to be undertaken to explain the new care model to patients. Many patients may be frustrated to learn that their conditions do not warrant immediate medical care in an ER setting. If there is no fast-track ER at the hospital where they are seeking treatment, they will be required to travel elsewhere. These patients may opt out of medical treatment altogether, which could drive up costs if their health care needs

aren't addressed expeditiously. Others may struggle with the cost of transportation. The public backlash could be significant.

6. Politicians and policy makers will have to take a potentially unpopular stance. The poor and underinsured are the highest abusers of ER care. No politician wants to touch an issue that could restrict care for the poor despite the fact that our current system has made considerable effort to redirect these patients to the alternate options that are available right now.

So the patients keep coming, the costs keep rising, and the finger-pointing continues its cycle of circular senselessness.

Health care: We have a problem.

CHAPTER 1

HEALTH CARE PRIMER: UNDERSTANDING HEALTH CARE'S UNIQUE LANGUAGE

Health care, like any other industry, has its own vocabulary, acronyms, and terms. I've highlighted some key terms that are used regularly in this book. These are not technical definitions. I've outlined layman's descriptions, and I emphasize the aspects of each of these areas that most relate to the topics in this book.

Much of the source data for my research was provided by governmental agencies. It can be difficult to weed through, but there is an absolute treasure trove of information available, should you be so inclined to review it. Other nonprofit organizations offer excellent industry summaries and data compilations. Some great sources for health care information include the Centers for Medicare and Medicaid Services, the U.S. Census Bureau, the World Health Organization, the Henry J. Kaiser Family Foundation, and the Commonwealth Fund.

DEFINITIONS

Providers. This is an all-encompassing term for the folks and institutions who provide care—from doctors and nurses to phlebotomists and pharmacists. The term also refers to the location of the care, meaning that hospitals and clinics are considered providers. Basically, any entity that gets paid to deliver health care is called a provider.

Payers. Whoever is paying for the care. So that would be insurance companies and public insurance programs like Medicare and Medicaid. If you pay out of pocket for an elective surgery, you're the payer.

Primary Care Provider. Primary care providers (PCPs) provide services for a patient's basic health care needs. If you get a physical, you'll see a primary care provider. When you go to a clinic, you'll see a primary care provider. Doctors can be primary care providers, but so can registered nurses (RNs) and physician assistants (PAs). Regulations are loosening regarding the authorized functions of non-physician primary caregivers due to a shortage of primary care doctors. Depending on the activity and the state, nurses and other primary care providers can conduct exams independently and prescribe certain medications.

Specialist. A physician who has advanced training in a specific area of medicine such as surgery (we all know what that is), cardiology (medical care related to the heart), orthopedics (care related to bones, joints), dermatology (the skin), etc.

Medicaid. The public health program for low-income Americans. Low-income senior citizens who cannot pay the costs not covered by Medicare may also qualify for Medicaid, making them dual-eligible beneficiaries.

Medicare. The public health program providing insurance for people aged sixty-five and older, younger people with selected disabilities, and individuals with end-stage renal disease.

Inpatient versus Outpatient. Inpatient care is delivered to individuals who are admitted to a hospital and stay for twenty-four hours or longer. Patients who can go home in less than twenty-four hours after being treated in a hospital are outpatients. There are some interpretations based on whether a patient has spent time in the emergency room under observation, but the twenty-four-hour metric is the simplest way to differentiate these patients.

Obese versus Overweight. Healthy (and unhealthy) weights for individuals are measured as a function of Body Mass Index, or BMI. BMI is an individual's weight in kilograms divided by the square of his or her height measured in meters. Per the Centers for Disease Control, if your BMI is 25 or more but less than 30, you are considered overweight. If your BMI is 30 or greater, you are considered obese.

Premium. The monthly payment an individual pays to an insurer for health insurance.

Co-Pay. An amount a patient is responsible for paying to a provider under an insurance plan. Co-pays vary by the type of coverage and by the service the patient accesses. Some plans may waive co-pays to primary care doctors, and most plans require a higher co-pay to see a specialist than to see a PCP.

Deductible. Similar to car insurance, this is the amount an individual must pay out of pocket before the insurance company will pay for certain aspects of coverage.

Elective. A procedure or test that is recommended by a provider but is not urgent. Patients can put off elective procedures, like knee replacements or cataract surgery, for months or even years. Yet in many cases, a condition not addressed by an elective procedure can worsen to the point that it becomes urgent. Patients are counseled to follow provider advice related to the recommended timelines for completing elective procedures.

ACRONYMS

ACA/Obamacare. Affordable Care Act. Officially called the Patient Protection and Affordable Care Act, this is President Barack Obama's signature legislation passed in 2010. Its intent was to provide all Americans with affordable health care coverage.

AHA. The American Hospital Association. This is the main lobbying group for hospitals in America that produces proprietary research and reports about the industry. The AHA's key goal of late is to figure out how to make sure hospitals can get paid as much as possible given the cost crunch impacting the industry.

AMA. The American Medical Association. This is the premier trade organization for physicians. It is the go-to resource for the medical community's view on clinical treatments and their relationship to policy. The AMA wants to make sure that no politician tells a doctor how to do his or her job.

CBO. The Congressional Budget Office. This nonpartisan group conducts economic impact analyses on proposed legislation. Lawmakers rely on the CBO's work to help them understand the short- and long-term financial impact of policy proposals across multiple industries.

CDC. Centers for Disease Control and Prevention. CDC is a component of the Department of Health and Human Services, but it is headquartered in Atlanta, not Washington, D.C. The CDC tracks disease, tries to find cures, and protects the nation against health threats.

CMS. The Centers for Medicare and Medicaid Services. I have no idea why it's not called CMMS, but that wouldn't be the first thing I don't understand about the organization. This federal agency is part of the Department of Health and Human Services and has the awesome responsibility of administering the major public health programs in America.

EMR. Electronic medical record. Also known as an EHR, or electronic health record. This technology is used to house medical and demographic information about a patient's health history. EMRs also support billing and payment functions and have modules customized for specific clinical departments such as surgery, radiology, and pharmacy. Common EMRs used by hospitals are those developed by Cerner, Epic, and Allscripts.

HDHP. High-deductible health plan. An insurance plan with a low monthly premium but a higher than average deductible. These plans are attractive for healthy Americans who do not expect to incur significant health care expenses.

PRIVATE INSURANCE

Private insurance, also known as commercial insurance, refers to health insurance coverage provided through many employers or bought directly from insurance companies by consumers. About half of all Americans get their health insurance from their employer, and another 7% buy it outright. Private insurance spending accounts for about a third, or approximately $1.1 trillion, of health care dollars spent in America.

Most commercial health insurance companies operate with the same business model. An insurer acts as a middleman between the patient (referred to as a member or an enrollee) and the provider (the doctor, hospital, clinic). The member contracts with the insurer for a twelve-month period. The member agrees to pay the insurer a monthly premium, which can run several hundred dollars but can be over $1,000. The member also agrees to pay different amounts of money for access to different goods and services.

Most plans require the member to pay a flat fee, called a deductible, before the insurance company will start paying for the member's health care per the contract. The deductible is typically several thousand dollars but can be over $10,000. Between the premium and deductible payments, many policyholders can spend well over $10,000 a year if they require significant medical care.

The insurer agrees to provide a select set of services, such as doctor visits, tests, surgeries, hospitalizations, or physical therapy. The insurer makes arrangements with providers to perform these services for their members. Members must use these contracted providers in order for their care to be covered by the plan. The insurer may have specific rules that a member must follow in order to access care, such as the need for a referral from one doctor in order to see another. Some insurers can deny care if they deem it experimental or if the type of care is not covered under the terms of the contract.

Health insurers function like other insuring agents. They seek to minimize risk by spreading potentially high-cost accounts over many other lower-cost accounts. Health insurers want as many healthy members as possible on their plans because these individuals do not require significant amounts of service. Insurers can use more of the healthy contingent's financial contributions toward funding the care required by sicker enrollees. Remaining funds are used to operate the insurer's business, are reinvested in the company, and/or drop to the bottom line as profit.

IMPACT OF THE AFFORDABLE CARE ACT

The implementation of the Affordable Care Act rattled the consumer health insurance market because it challenged insurers' abilities to satisfy the law's requirements and still provide care that was affordable. The law has many components which have been implemented either fully, partially, or reversed through Supreme Court verdicts, executive orders, and other legislative efforts.

The plans are mostly sold through ACA "marketplaces" or "exchanges," which consolidate a market's offerings in one online community. This is why ACA plans are sometimes called marketplace or exchange plans. Some states have created their own exchanges where their residents can shop for plans. Consumers whose states do not have an exchange can find offerings on the federal healthcare.gov website.

The legislation affects health insurance plans offered to consumers, which is less than 10% of the population. Yet for reasons described below, the ACA is one of the factors contributing to instability and uncertainty in both the public and private insurance markets.

The most popular element of ACA, at least as far as consumers are concerned, is the prohibition of insurers to be able to reject applicants based on a preexisting condition. While the provision has opened up the market to those previously denied care, it has also been the major driver in cost increases. Individuals with preexisting conditions may require thousands, even millions of dollars to cover the cost of their care. Since insurers don't know whether very ill individuals will sign up for their plans, they can't estimate the risk level associated with their potential members. That, in turn, makes it hard for them to set prices. As a result, insurers may overprice to mitigate their risk.

The ACA also requires that marketplace plans provide *ten essential benefits*. These benefits include services such as hospital care, outpatient care, rehabilitation, and mental health services whether potential buyers want them or not. The ten essential benefits requirement makes the plans more expensive because of the broad coverage that must be offered. Only insurers with sophisticated contracting expertise and comprehensive industry contacts are able to cobble together the comprehensive suite of services required by law. That makes it harder for smaller insurers to offer ACA plans.

The ACA included provisions that changed the income qualification for Medicaid, thereby enabling more low-income Americans to enroll in the program. The ACA provided federal funding to cover most of the cost of the expansion, but some states objected to expanding a program they considered inefficient. Some believed that the ACA's de facto mandate to add dollars to their state budgets to pay for their portion of the expansion was federal overreach. Legal arguments ensued as more than twenty states initially rejected the Medicaid expansion requirement of the ACA.[1]

The issue went all the way to the Supreme Court in the case the *National Federation of Independent Business (NFIB) v. Sebelius*.[2] In June of 2012, the Supreme Court ostensibly ruled that the expansion was voluntary. Since then, more states have expanded their Medicaid programs, although some have negotiated to add their own state-specific terms, such as work or volunteer requirements for enrollees. At print, seventeen[3] states had still declined participation in the expansion authorized by ACA (although one could argue that Maine should also be included in the count, as its adaption is currently hung up in an intrastate legal battle).

The *National Federation of Independent Business (NFIB) v. Sebelius* ruling determined that a separate but also contentious aspect of the law, the individual mandate, was constitutional. As noted earlier, the individual mandate is an aspect of the law that requires every American to buy health insurance or face a financial penalty. Despite the Court's opinion, many objected to the individual mandate because the plans that Americans were required to buy were arguably bloated by the ten essential benefits requirement and too expensive because of the high number of sick individuals in the market.

In response to these concerns, Congress eliminated the individual mandate as part of the Tax Cuts and Jobs Act of 2017. Many are concerned that healthy Americans will now opt out of buying insurance altogether, leaving those who remain in the pool of applicants sicker and thus more expensive to insure.

While the ACA only directly impacts the approximately twenty million Americans buying ACA plans, the legislation indirectly affects the rest of us. First, the ACA allowed for government-funded subsidies paid to insurers to cover the cost of insurance premiums that were too expensive for low-income shoppers. Taxpayers foot the bill for these subsidies, for which 85% of the buyers on the healthcare. gov website were eligible in 2016.[4] The Trump administration moved to eliminate some of these subsidies in 2017, although negotiations with insurers are ongoing. Without the subsidies, the ACA insurance market would be on the verge of collapse.

Without the individual mandate and with the threat of eliminating the subsidies, health insurance on the marketplace will continue to be too expensive for many to afford. When the uninsured require medical care, they put themselves at risk of financial ruin. One recent study indicated that seven out of ten uninsured individuals who required trauma care in the ER were left with financially catastrophic medical bills.[5]

If individuals can't pay for their care, then it's up to the rest of the health care system to fund it. That means that other Americans indirectly pay for the care through taxes, donations, and increases in health care costs throughout the system. Between 2013 (when ACA went into effect) and 2016, the price of family premiums offered through employer-sponsored plans increased 11%.[6]

But many more costs were shifted to employees through a dramatic rise in deductibles. From 2011 to 2016, the cumulative increase in single coverage (nonfamily) deductibles was 63%.[7] And between 2010 and 2017, the number of Americans enrolled in high-deductible health plans (HDHP) doubled to over twenty-one million people.[8] An HDHP offers a lower monthly premium in exchange for a higher-priced deductible. These plans are advantageous for healthy Americans, but if these members require medical care, they'll foot much more of the bill with an HDHP than they would with more traditional insurance. While these increases cannot be solely attributed to the ACA, there's no doubt that the effects of the legislation are being felt financially to some degree by all Americans.

INSURERS' COST CONTROL STRATEGIES

Regardless of what transpires with ACA, the cost of health care in America is increasing. Health outcomes in America have been declining, as evidenced by our increasing rates of obesity, chronic disease, and drops in life expectancy. As more Americans become less healthy, insurers have to figure out a way to provide for care while remaining financially viable. There are several mechanisms insurers can and have used to make sure they maintain their profitability.

Insurers have been passing on more of the cost of care to members. As noted previously, premiums and deductibles have been rising, which provides more revenue to the insurer. More and more individuals are enrolling in high-deductible health plans. HDHP can be good for insurers because patients with these plans use fewer health care services than individuals not enrolled in HDHPs. For example, HDHP enrollees use fewer inpatient services and are much more likely to postpone elective care because they'll have to pay for it out of their own pockets. That means the cost of paying for the care for HDHP enrollees can be less for the insurer, making these individuals more attractive, financially.

The insurers can also make it difficult or challenging to access care. Some plans require a referral from a primary care doctor for specialty care, and this extra step can be a deterrent for an individual who does not have a life-threatening condition. Even plans without this restriction may institute access hurdles, such as requiring in-office doctor visits to review lab work, additional tests to confirm a diagnosis, or other evaluations that could lead to a delay or denial of care under the terms of the plan's contract.

Alternatively, insurers can put up roadblocks to paying providers by forcing them to comply with detailed terms of payment. This is a significant problem for providers because the terms of service can vary from one insurer to another. For example, one insurer could deny payment for any claim not submitted within forty-five days of service. Another insurer may need the claim within thirty days. Insurers can also dictate the mode of communication between the provider and the payer. Some payers have dedicated websites that providers must log in to. And believe it or not, many insurers still communicate with providers via fax.

Some insurers require providers to pre-authorize certain tests and procedures before performing them. It's sort of like the doctor has to ask permission from the insurance company before they can do their job. Pre-authorizations add both administrative and clinical costs to the system. Administrative costs increase because of the time it takes to secure the approval from the insurer and then communicate with the patient. In some cases, patients have to schedule follow-up appointments with the provider after the authorization has been approved. This is inconvenient and costly for the patient and the provider. Some patients don't come back, and then the insurer doesn't have to pay for their care. In a worst-case scenario, the delay in care caused by the pre-authorization can cause a health condition to worsen. This is a less desirable outcome for both the insurer and the patient, but it is a by-product of this burdensome requirement.

PUBLIC INSURANCE

Medicare and Medicaid are the two largest public insurance programs. These programs, as well as the Children's Health Insurance Program (CHIP), which covers low-income qualified children, are administered by CMS. Veterans Affairs (VA) is another public program, which provides lifetime health care benefits to qualified veterans and their families. The VA is considered a "closed system" because the majority of its services are delivered via its own separate hospitals, physicians, and administration. Health care provided for the Department of Defense for active military is also considered public health care.

MEDICARE

In 2016, the United States spent $672 billion on Medicare. The program consists of multiple "parts" that correspond to different aspects of the delivery system.[9] Medicare Part A is for inpatient hospital stays, skilled nursing, home care, and hospice care. Part B is for care typically delivered in the outpatient environment. Physician office visits, ambulance service, certain drugs, and durable medical equipment (known as DME and includes items like wheelchairs and walkers) are covered under Part B. Medicare Part D covers many prescription drugs.

Medicare is the single largest payer (insurer) in the United States. As a result, Medicare wields significant power in setting health policy and standards. Most health care facilities must satisfy clinical and operational regulations established by Medicare in order to receive payment for enrollees in the program. As will be discussed later in this book, Medicare also establishes categories and classifications for myriad clinical episodes, from a simple X-ray to a coronary artery bypass graft (known as a CABG and oftentimes performed as open-heart surgery). Other insurers are highly influenced by these codes and guidelines and often default to Medicare's rulings. For example, Medicare may approve payment for a certain type of surgery to be conducted in an outpatient environment. Other insurers are almost certain to follow Medicare's lead and will adjust their payment schedules accordingly.

Medicare revenue is derived from a number of sources. In 2017, general revenue (money in the coffers of the U.S. Treasury, which got there from sources like taxes and interest) accounted for 41% of funding. Payroll taxes (a 2.9% tax split equally between employers and employees at 1.45% each) contributed 37%. Premium payments, or what enrollees pay out of pocket, were 14%, and the remainder was funded through other sources such as a tax on Social Security payments and interest from the Medicare Trust Fund.[10]

Between 2007 and 2016, Medicare spending per capita grew between 4% and 8% every year. The spending issue is going to become more problematic because the baby boomer population is aging into the program. They're staying alive longer, which is great for them but terrible for budgeters and taxpayers. By 2050, the population over the age of sixty-five is expected to be twice of what it was in 2012.[11] One projection indicates that if Medicare outlays continue on pace, the Medicare Trust Fund (mentioned above) will be insolvent in 2026.[12]

Medicare does not cover all the costs for the different parts of its program. Enrollees are responsible for co-pays, deductibles, and portions of different kinds of care. Furthermore, there is no limit on out-of-pocket expenses for traditional Medicare coverage. (Medicare Advantage plans, described below, do have a cap.) In other words, if a Medicare enrollee is hospitalized for a serious illness, then he or she is responsible for the uncovered portion of care—which could be hundreds of thousands of dollars. On top of that, Medicare does not cover dental, vision, hearing, or long-term care. This is why most Medicare beneficiaries need some sort of supplemental coverage.

An increasingly popular way for Medicare beneficiaries to supplement their coverage is through a Medicare Advantage plan (also known as Medicare Part C).[13] Medicare Advantage plans are offered by commercial insurers and cover all the costs of Part A and Part B. Some plans may offer coverage for Part D (the drugs) too. Secondary insurance can also be provided through Medicare Supplement Insurance (Medigap).[14] These plans cover what is not covered under Medicare Parts A and B. Separate insurance would be required for prescription drug coverage not provided through Part D.

These few paragraphs only scratch the surface of the complexities of the program. Despite its unwieldy construct, Medicare is wildly popular with seniors. It provides them with the security of health care coverage that they have been promised by the government throughout their adult lives. Even better for seniors is the fact that they're getting a great deal. That's because the amount that current Medicare recipients have contributed to the system over their lifetimes is much less than the cost of the care they're receiving.[15]

MEDICAID

Medicaid provides public health coverage for certain low-income individuals and families. In 2016, $572 billion was spent on the program. Medicaid is a collaboration between federal and state governments. The feds pay about 60% of Medicaid costs, and the states pick up the rest. Given the variability of state regulations, the program is administered differently from state to state.

Over 40% of Medicaid enrollees are children, and they account for less than 20% of the program's costs. About half the births in America are funded by Medicaid. That means that half of the babies born are coming into families that are financially challenged. Children born into low-income families are more likely to have lower levels of education, lower levels of income, and poorer health. These individuals face obstacles in caring for themselves and, subsequently, their families.

Many Americans view Medicaid as "health insurance for the poor." Yet a considerable component of program dollars goes toward those who are aged and/or have disabilities. The aged and disabled account for about 20% of enrollees. About a third of Medicaid spending goes toward the disabled. Approximately 15% of Medicaid dollars fund care for so-called dual-eligible individuals: the poor (however it is defined by the government) and the aged (who are also covered by Medicare). Together, the aged and disabled account for about half of the costs in the program.[16]

For qualified dual-eligible enrollees, the cost for nursing home care is covered by Medicaid. Nursing home care runs about $80,000 a year per patient. Yet Medicaid does not automatically cover home health costs, which can be dramatically lower than nursing home costs. Advances in technology have enabled many more Americans to age in place (i.e., stay in their homes), which is oftentimes a more attractive option than a nursing home. The program has yet to changes its policies and authorize payment for aging-in-place strategies.[17]

Ironically, Medicaid is touted for its so-called efficiency. According to CMS, "Medicaid is the most efficient health coverage program we have, covering people at lower cost than commercial insurance coverage or even Medicare."[18] Statements like this make an uninformed reader believe that the program should be expanded because of its low-cost model.

Unfortunately, this belief ignores one of the major problems with the Medicaid program: It significantly under-reimburses providers. On average, hospitals are paid only eighty-eight cents for every dollar they spend on Medicaid beneficiaries, and many facilities are paid less than that.[19] Primary care doctors are probably the most impacted, and low reimbursement is a major reason that America has a shortage of primary care doctors. A shortage of primary care doctors has been identified as a major problem for care access and quality, particularly in rural areas around the country.[20, 21]

CONCLUSION

The American health care system is capable of providing some of the best clinical care in the world. Unfortunately, this level of world-class service does not characterize the delivery and payment systems.

Countries across the globe are seeking American technology and ideas, but no one wants to replicate the way we deliver care to our citizens.

We are a consumer-driven society, and our patience for slow adaptation is minimal. So many of the industry's practices and behaviors are out of sync with what the average American expects in terms of service, quality, and price transparency. Case in point: why do we have to fill out paperwork on a clipboard every time we go to a doctor when, in the same amount of time, we can buy tickets to a movie, shop for our dinner, and order up a ride from our phones?

As dysfunctional as our system is, it could be a lot worse. In India, poor sanitation contributes to the country's overburdened, underfunded health care system. Diarrhea is the third leading cause of death.[22] Some may be surprised to learn that one of Africa's major problems is air quality. It's gotten so bad that poor air quality contributed to more premature deaths on the continent than the effects of unsafe water or malnutrition.[23]

While it is easy to critique the American system, which I have done and will continue to do throughout this book, we must appreciate the monumental contributions made by those before us to bring us to where we are today. With over 325 million diverse citizens in our country, we will never have a system that provides everything that everyone wants or needs. Yet we can certainly improve what we have today. The change will take patience, cooperation, and the continued supply of bright ideas and solutions from our American family.

CHAPTER 2

THE MONEY: WHERE IT ALL GOES

America: land of the free, home of the iPhone, inventor of the automobile, the zipper, the laser, and a zillion other paradigm-shifting products. We champion ideas. We're obsessed with inventing, disrupting, and innovating our way out of the status quo. We love risk-taking, deal-making, nose-to-the-grindstone, hard-working personalities. We celebrate and reward those who transform concepts into new realities. But despite our ambitious spirit, no one has been able to successfully reform—or more importantly, transform—what is arguably the most critical aspect of American society: the health care system.

In 2016, the United States spent $3.3 trillion on health care.[1] The $3.3 trillion is an aggregation of dollars expended across our economy, meaning that it's not just what was distributed by the federal government. It estimates the funds spent by all levels of government, insurance companies, and individuals on a comprehensive range of goods and services, including hospital care, outpatient care, drugs, medical equipment, nursing home care, and over-the-counter health-related expenses.

The following chart breaks down the source of payment for the $3.3 trillion in health care expenditures in 2016.[2]

CHART 1. 2016 NATIONAL HEALTH EXPENDITURES *($3.3 TRILLION TOTAL)*
BY SOURCE OF PAYMENT *($ BILLIONS)*

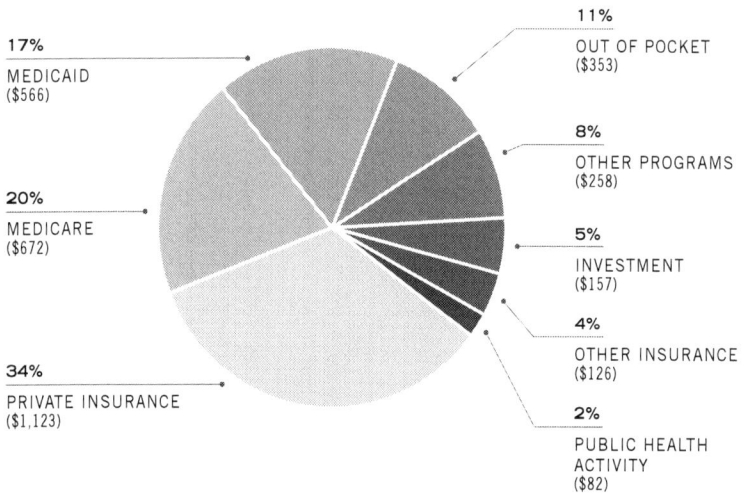

11%
OUT OF POCKET
($353)

17%
MEDICAID
($566)

8%
OTHER PROGRAMS
($258)

20%
MEDICARE
($672)

5%
INVESTMENT
($157)

4%
OTHER INSURANCE
($126)

34%
PRIVATE INSURANCE
($1,123)

2%
PUBLIC HEALTH
ACTIVITY
($82)

Totals do not sum to 100 due to rounding.

About half the dollars in the system, or over $1.6 trillion, were spent by federal, state, and local governments. Most of the money is expended by Medicare or Medicaid. The Veterans Administration, CHIP (Children's Health Insurance Program), and a host of other programs are also included in this governmental grouping under the categories Other Programs and Other Insurance.[3] About one in every three dollars is spent by a private insurance company.

That translates to over $1.1 trillion spent by companies like United-Healthcare, Anthem, and Aetna.

Ten percent, or about $353 billion, is spent on out-of-pocket expenses. This includes categories such as co-insurance payments and deductibles that individuals pay for covered health care-related expenses. Other expenditures not covered by an insurer, such as chiropractic services, acupuncture, or elective procedures, are included, too. Retail expenditures, like over-the-counter drugs such as aspirin and allergy medications, also roll up into this figure.[4]

About $157 billion, or 5% of the spend, is spent on research and investment. This covers government-funded research programs, grants, and new buildings. It does not include the research and development that is funded by pharmaceutical companies for the development of new drugs.

Finally, $82 billion, or 2% of our health care spending, is spent on public health. Any American, whether enrolled in private insurance or in a public program, is a beneficiary of public health dollars. This money is spent on education about health-related issues. Anti-smoking campaigns, programs to stop bullying, and advice about nutrition and vaccines are the types of spending included in this category.

HEALTH CARE SOLUTIONS TARGETED TO HALF THE POPULATION CAN'T TRANSFORM THE SYSTEM

It's important to note that although the government spends about half the health care dollars in America, the money isn't spent on half of all Americans. Public health care covers only about a third of Americans (those enrolled in Medicare, Medicaid, and other public programs). The following chart outlines the percentage of Americans who get their health insurance through different mechanisms.[5]

CHART 2. 2016 % TOTAL POPULATION
BY TYPE OF INSURANCE COVERAGE

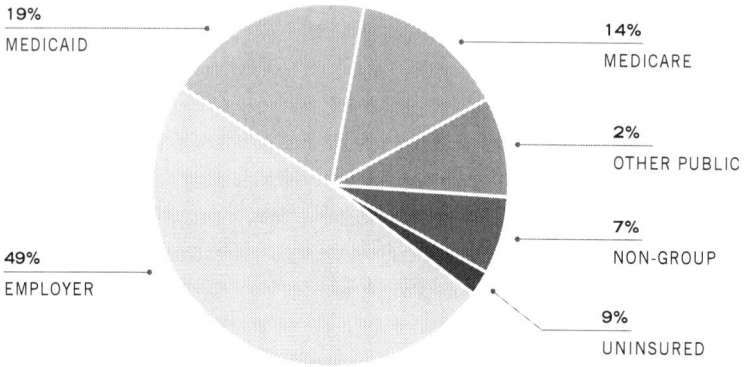

19%
MEDICAID

14%
MEDICARE

2%
OTHER PUBLIC

7%
NON-GROUP

49%
EMPLOYER

9%
UNINSURED

Well over half, or 56%, of Americans have health insurance that is provided by private or commercial insurance (see Employer and Non-Group). About 49% of that 56% get their insurance through plans offered by their employers. The Non-Group category represents 7% of the population who buy insurance on the open market through ACA health care exchanges, directly from insurers, or from brokers. These private-pay individuals represent over half the population, but as noted in Chart 1, use only about a third of the health care dollars that are spent in America.[6]

What's interesting to note here is the inverse relationship between public and private insurance enrollment and health care spending. We spend more per person on public health than we do on private insurance.

CHART 3. 2016 COVERAGE SPENDING COMPARISON
BY TYPE OF INSURANCE COVERAGE AND
TOTAL HEALTH EXPENDITURES

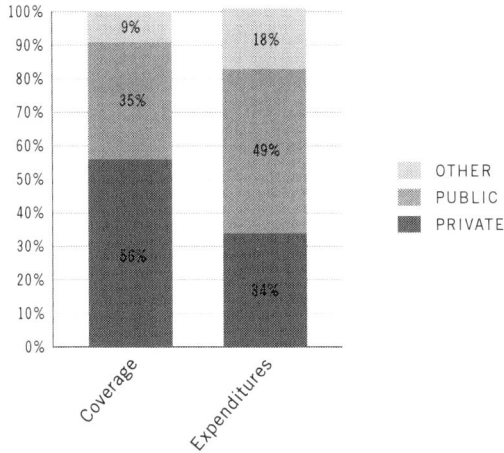

Totals do not sum to 100 due to rounding.

There are a variety of reasons for this imbalance in spending. The most important factor relates to the patient base that's being covered by each of the programs. Enrollees in private insurance are typically healthier and wealthier than those served in public programs. Higher income levels correlate to higher levels of education, and both of these factors correlate to better health status. Healthier folks use fewer services and therefore cost less to treat.

Another reason is that the majority of an individual's health care costs occur at the end of life—when patients are enrolled in Medicare. That factor alone significantly impacts the higher per-person spend on public versus private insurance. If you factor in that the Medicaid population is, by definition, less wealthy than other Americans, it follows that it is characterized by a lower level of education about health and disease prevention issues. That's why the health status of these groups will skew more poorly than average. It's understandable that we'd be spending more on public health programs than on commercial care for them.

This relationship becomes important when we talk about the impact that certain programs could have on changing the health care industry. Those who are privately insured are healthier, more educated, and—of critical importance to investors looking to fund companies that are attempting to transform the industry—have more money to spend than other constituents. This market could be great for so-called disruptive solutions, given that the spend by private insurers is over a trillion dollars a year, and this group represents well over half of Americans. But unless the solutions targeted toward the private-pay majority can also be adapted by the publicly insured, they can't be disruptive. These innovations are potentially profitable, but they're not transformative.

RISING HEALTH CARE COSTS AND FISCAL RESPONSIBILITY

Here is an interesting factoid: The $3.3 trillion spent on health care yearly in the United States roughly approximates the GDP of Germany,[7] one of the most prosperous economies in the world. To give you some context about the challenges associated with effectively managing a chunk of money that big, consider that Angela Merkel, Germany's long-time chancellor, has a PhD in quantum chemistry. It helps to have brains at the top.

Yet even the smartest of people, the most compassionate of heart, the most innovative in spirit are having trouble not just managing our current health care spending, but also tamping down its growth. Health care spending in America has been increasing at a steady clip. Each year from 2007 to 2016, overall spending has increased somewhere between 3% and 6%.

The following chart shows the increase in total health care expenditures as well as the per capita costs over the ten-year period leading up to 2016. Spending increased over a trillion dollars from $2.3

trillion in 2007 to $3.3 trillion in 2016. Over that same period, the per capita spending jumped from $7,626 to $10,364.

CHART 4. 2007–2016 NATIONAL HEALTH EXPENDITURES
TOTAL / COST PER CAPITA

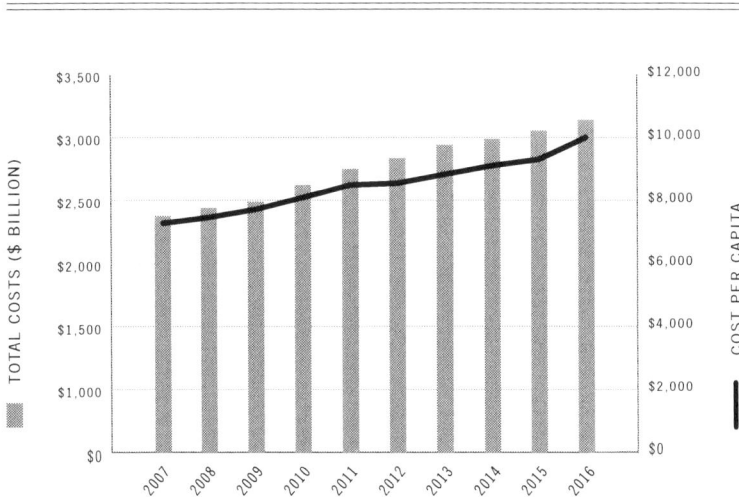

We should expect health care costs to increase over time because the size of our population has been increasing. If there are more people, more will be spent on health care (assuming the rate of spend holds steady). However, we're not only spending more money in aggregate, we're spending more money per person.

By way of comparison, the budget for the federal government was $3.9 trillion in 2016. Health care spending, at $3.3 trillion, was only 15% less than what was spent on the federal programs overseen by the folks in Washington.

The following chart shows the categories of spending in the 2016 federal budget as broken out by the nonpartisan Congressional Budget Office (CBO).[8] As noted earlier, Medicaid is funded by the federal and state governments. Chart 5 only shows the federal government's spend, or $368 billion out of the entire $566 billion spent on Medicaid in 2016.

CHART 5. 2016 FEDERAL BUDGET SPENDING *($3.9 TRILLION TOTAL)*
BY CATEGORY *($ BILLIONS)*

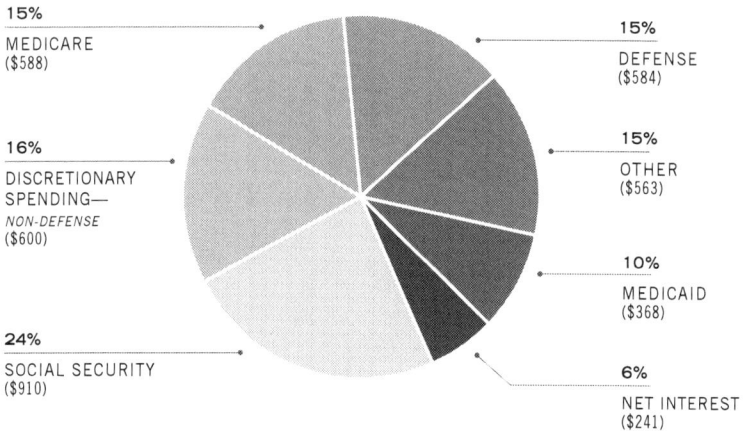

15%
MEDICARE
($588)

15%
DEFENSE
($584)

16%
DISCRETIONARY
SPENDING—
NON-DEFENSE
($600)

15%
OTHER
($563)

10%
MEDICAID
($368)

24%
SOCIAL SECURITY
($910)

6%
NET INTEREST
($241)

Totals do not sum to 100 due to rounding.

Further, the Medicare figure, at $588 billion, is less than total Medicare expenditures of $672 billion noted in Chart 1. The difference can largely be attributed to the fact that the CBO's total is only looking at what the government had to spend. Any premiums and payments that Medicare enrollees pay out of pocket are not included in the $588 billion, because those payments were made by individuals, not by the feds. Those dollars are, however, included in the $672 billion Medicare portion of the National Health Expenditures for 2016 noted in Chart 1.

Medicare and Medicaid combined total about a quarter of federal spending. Social Security spending is at the same level. In other words, half of all the dollars spent by the federal government are going to these three entitlement programs. Costs for other health care expenditures, such as veteran's benefits and other health-related programs, are embedded in Discretionary Spending (Non-Defense) and Other.

HEALTH CARE SPENDING HAS CREATED A SERIOUS FINANCIAL CRISIS

The federal government spent $3.9 trillion in 2016, but it only collected $3.3 trillion (which is, coincidentally, the same amount we spend on health care). Herein lies a serious problem. *We aren't collecting enough money to pay for what the federal government spends right now.* A significant portion of what the federal government spends is on health care. If we don't bring in enough dollars, we need to cut spending. But spending on health care is rising. Not surprisingly, the Congressional Budget Office has concluded that a primary driver of our growing national debt is Medicare spending.[9]

We could keep the spending level as it is and simply raise revenues—i.e., taxes. But the tax overhaul passed in November 2017 may create just the opposite effect. A key aspect of the legislation was the reduction of the corporate tax rate. In 2016, when the corporate tax rate for large companies was 35% to 38%, $300 billion in corporate taxes were collected. The law drops the rate to a flat 21%. As a result, many believe less than $300 billion will be collected from this critical tax source in the coming years.

Others believe that the tax overhaul will stimulate the economy. Additional revenues would be collected from categories such as taxes on increased consumer spending, real estate taxes from the purchase of new homes, and taxes on spending conducted by new businesses as well as the associated taxes on their incomes. Some are hoping that U.S. companies with headquarters located abroad will move back to the United States, thereby adding to the taxes collected from corporations. It's hard to know. At best, one can hope that revenues won't go down.

SPENDING BEYOND OUR MEANS

If we keep spending more and more on health care, and we're not expecting commensurate increases in revenues, our nation is going to find itself in dangerous financial territory. Right now, our federal debt, which is the accumulated amount of money our government owes due to deficit spending and other financial obligations, is over $21 trillion. It's the single largest debt load of any country in the world. But then again, we are the largest economy in the world (by some measures), so we need to keep these figures in perspective.

A metric that economists like to use when considering if a country is overspending is the deficit-to-GDP ratio. That compares a single year's overspending (deficit) to the nation's economic output, or Gross Domestic Product (GDP). If the percentage crosses -3%, then the government is overspending. This figure is used by the European Union as a means to check the economic status of member nations. Germany's ratio in 2017 was 0.7%. That means they didn't have a deficit. That same year, the United Kingdom's ratio was -3.6% while the United States' ratio was -3.4%.[10]

Going back to Chart 5, we note that 6% of federal government spending was on interest. Interest rates have been low, so economists don't panic so much about our debt. Yet at some point, interest rates are going to go up. The government bonds that the federal government sells to investors in order to bring in the extra cash we need to cover our costs will have to be sold at higher interest rates. That means that when the government pays back investors, it has to pay them back at a higher rate. Such a cycle increases our spending, which, in turn, makes it harder to bring down the debt. It simply isn't financially responsible to keep spending.

POOR OUTCOMES FOR A FIRST-WORLD NATION

Our health care spending is at fiscally irresponsible levels, yet the system is severely hampered in its efforts to reduce costs because

Americans are so unhealthy. It's a vicious cycle. We spend money on health care because our society is so sick. Yet one would think that by spending so much money, we should be healthier. We're not.

In fact, we're starting to live shorter lives. Life expectancy dropped in 2015 for the first time in decades when it dipped to 78.8 from 78.9 in 2014.[11] The drop was small, and many had hoped that the figure was an anomaly. But in 2016, it dropped again, to 78.6.[12]

Compared to the rest of the world, life expectancy in America isn't all that great. The World Health Organization (WHO) ranks countries based on this measure and many other factors. Out of 183 other countries, we rank 34th in life expectancy.[13] The majority of industrialized nations rank ahead of us. Japan ranked number one.

CHART 6. 2016 LIFE EXPECTANCY AT BIRTH
BY COUNTRY

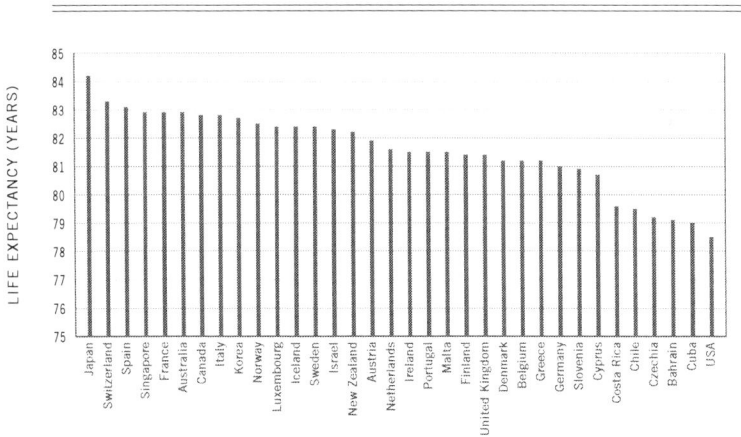

Similarly, the maternal mortality rate, or the rate at which mothers die as a result of complications from pregnancy or childbirth, has been increasing in our country. From 2000 to 2014, the maternal death rate increased from nineteen to twenty-four deaths per 100,000 live births.[14]

By 2015, it was 26.4, the worst in the developed world.[15] Issues contributing to the increase include poor access to care in rural communities, inconsistent clinical care quality, and the health of the mothers.

The rising rate of obesity in America is a particular concern. Excess weight can challenge a woman's ability to handle the strain of carrying and delivering a baby, which can create complications such as preeclampsia (high blood pressure that can damage the mother's organs, cause premature birth, or require an emergency Caesarian section).

The increase in opioid-related deaths is a significant factor in the decline in American life expectancy.[16] Between 1999 and 2016, over 350,000 people died of opioid-related drug overdoses.[17] The rate of opioid deaths increased five times over the period between 1999 and 2016.[18] Historically problematic street drugs like heroin, legally prescribed painkillers like Vicodin, and powerful synthetic opioids like fentanyl were to blame for these deaths. Sometimes they were taken together.

Lawsuits against drug companies that produce opioids are piling up, and the Justice Department got involved in early 2018. The cases contain allegations relating to how drug companies misinformed or misled providers about the addictive qualities of the drugs. If doctors knew that the drugs were so powerful—the supposition is—they would have been more careful with how they were prescribing them to patients. Cases like these have been brought before. In 2007, OxyContin producer Purdue Pharma agreed to pay $600 million in fines.[19]

But pharmaceutical companies can't and shouldn't shoulder all the blame for the drug use epidemic. Last I checked, Purdue Pharma didn't make heroin. There's something deeper and more troubling going on that's driving Americans' problems with addiction.

Cultural, economic, and clinical factors are all at play. Ultimately, addiction in any form reflects deep underlying mental health issues. Mental health problems have been stigmatized for generations. Many who need treatment refuse to accept the fact that they need help or are too ashamed to seek it out. Improving cultural awareness about mental health issues will continue to be an increasingly important factor in addressing this problem.

Improving cultural awareness is also going to be necessary to address our obesity problem. Obesity is one of the most critical health issues in America because of its relationship to health concerns like type 2 diabetes, heart disease, stroke, and certain types of cancer.[20] Not only are obese people more prone to develop health conditions, it also takes them longer to recover from treatments like surgery. These augmented health needs have financial consequences. Obese adults spend 42% more on direct health care expenses than those who are at a healthy weight.[21]

There seems to be an unfortunate disconnect between our perceptions about being overweight and the reality of the situation. As outlined in Chart 7, over the past few decades, the percentage of Americans who are classified as overweight or obese has grown.[22] Yet over the same period, the percentage of Americans who *think* they're overweight has fallen.[23]

CHART 7. AMERICANS' VIEWS ABOUT THEIR WEIGHT
SELECTED YEARS

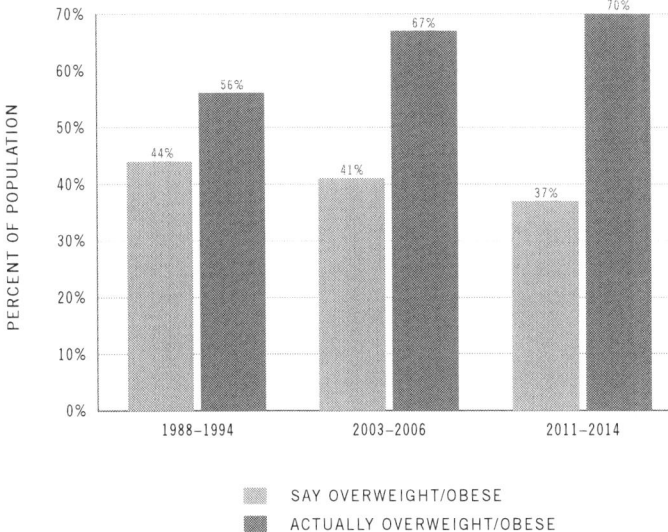

Bar chart. Y-axis: PERCENT OF POPULATION, from 0% to 70%. X-axis categories: 1988–1994, 2003–2006, 2011–2014.

- 1988–1994: SAY OVERWEIGHT/OBESE 44%, ACTUALLY OVERWEIGHT/OBESE 56%
- 2003–2006: SAY OVERWEIGHT/OBESE 41%, ACTUALLY OVERWEIGHT/OBESE 67%
- 2011–2014: SAY OVERWEIGHT/OBESE 37%, ACTUALLY OVERWEIGHT/OBESE 70%

Legend:
SAY OVERWEIGHT/OBESE
ACTUALLY OVERWEIGHT/OBESE

This is a bizarre phenomenon that can be partially explained by the "normalization" of obesity. This chart shows that the more people are exposed to others who are obese—i.e., as the rates of obesity rise—the more normal it seems. As a result, Americans seem less and less inclined to think they are overweight because more and more people around them are becoming heavier and heavier.

From a global standpoint, the United States is one of the most obese nations in the world. Out of the 35 member nations in the OECD (Organisation for Economic Co-operation and Development), the United States has the highest obesity rate for men and women.[24]

Obesity in children is also climbing. Since the 1970s, the number of obese children has tripled, and today, about one in five children is obese. Sadly, children who are obese are more likely to remain obese as adults.[25] These kids are prone to many of the same diseases as obese adults, and may also suffer bullying, which adds a serious psychological burden for them to bear along with the physical ramifications of being excessively overweight.

CONCLUSION

The evidence is clear. We're unhealthy, and being unhealthy drives up health care costs. Increasing health care costs are affecting governmental budgets at all levels. When the federal budget is exceeded, we need to borrow money. When we borrow money, our debt increases. When the federal debt gets too high, we spend more money paying it off when we should be using the money to invest in the American people.

Somehow, we need to come to terms with the fact that despite our nation's prodigious wealth, we cannot afford to pay for all the health care options available for every single American. A look back at how we got to this point of financial peril can help provide some perspectives so we can positively re-chart our future.

CHAPTER 3

A HISTORICAL VIEW OF HEALTH POLICY: HOW DID THINGS GET SO COMPLICATED?

"We are not disposed to grumble or overstate the evil condition
of the public physique; we wish to call attention to the fact how
easily most these deficiencies might be remedied. Our theory is that
America has mentality enough but needs a far nobler physique."[1]

This quote is from *Manly Health and Training: To Teach the Science of a Sound and Beautiful Body*, a recently rediscovered Walt Whitman manifesto written in 1858. This series of essays espouses an individual's responsibility to be in good health, and it is well worth reading because it was written before the Civil War. Back then, there was no Medicaid or Medicare. Antibiotics wouldn't come along for another fifty years.[2] Surgical procedures were barbaric at best. (Just watch the

"Battle of Atlanta Injuries" scene from *Gone with the Wind*, and you'll know exactly what I'm talking about.) With minimal social support, everyone had to be much more self-reliant than they are today. There simply were no other options.

Health care in America has evolved into an overly complicated, expensive, inefficient beast. Whitman would be rolling over in his grave if he had to log on to healthcare.gov or enroll in a Medicare Advantage plan. There's no question that there's a financial imperative to change how we're doing things. *Yet the change that's needed is so radical, it's almost impossible to fathom.* How did things get so complicated?

In this chapter I will provide a historical perspective of key moments in health care politics and policy. Combined with some trends and societal expectations about how the system should work, we, collectively, should be able to recalibrate what the health care system is supposed to do, what we want out of it, and what we should spend on it.

EARLY HISTORY

Many people date the first health insurance program to a group of Dallas, Texas, teachers. In 1929, a group of instructors with Baylor University contracted with a local hospital to prepay for a hospital stay, should they be hospitalized at some time in the future. They paid the hospital in increments, providing the facility with a steady revenue stream and the teachers with peace of mind.[3] During the same year, Blue Cross developed health insurance plans based off the Baylor model.[4]

Soon the concept began to spread, and things really took off in 1942. Millions of men were out of the workforce and on the battlefield, so to speak, during World War II. Because competition among available stateside workers was fierce, Congress was concerned about rising wages and their impact on the economy. So it passed the Stabilization Act in an effort to tamp down on wage hikes. With pay rates controlled, employers had to look for other means by which to attract employees. One option was to offer health insurance.

As the years passed, more employers worked with insurance companies to develop programs that covered the cost of selected health services for their employees and their families. Employers were encouraged further when Congress passed the Revenue Act of 1954, which allowed employers to exclude contributions to employee health plans from taxable income. The impact of this legislation is still in place today. One estimate indicates that the amount of tax revenue that could be collected if employer-sponsored health insurance benefits were taxed equates to about $260 billion a year.[5]

EVERYONE WAS DOING PRETTY WELL

If we take a look back to America's Golden Age, or the period after World War II prior to the recession in the 1970s, the payment model that was used by insurers to pay doctors and hospitals was fairly straightforward. Doctors and hospitals used what is called a fee-for-service (FFS) model, and it's still in use today. Providers charged rates that they considered appropriate for services they deemed medically necessary. Insurers set some standards and controls, but their rules had a nominal impact on the financial health of hospitals, doctors, and insurers. Everyone was doing pretty well. But then again, so was everyone else in 1960—at least with regard to health status. (Civil rights were another story.)

During those years, the population was healthier and younger than it is today. In 1960, the median age was just under thirty years old.[6] Less than 15% of the population was obese.[7] The demand for health care services was lower because there were fewer drugs on the market to prescribe, fewer types of surgeries being performed, and fewer people being covered.

Importantly, Americans' demographic homogeneity also kept costs down. Eighty-five percent of Americans were white.[8] About 90% identified as Christian.[9] Behaviors, both good and bad, of most Americans were similar. That made it simpler to identify health problems and easier to fix them because messaging needed to be tailored to one main group. As will be discussed later in this book, America's current cultural diversity makes public health much more challenging because of the significant variability in behaviors and values.

Nineteen sixty-five was a landmark year in American health care history. President Lyndon B. Johnson signed Medicare and Medicaid into law, creating national public health programs for the elderly and the needy. These programs were welcomed by many Americans when they were initiated. They were also very small. In 1970, National Health Expenditures as a percentage of GDP was 6.9%.[10] In 2016, it was 17.9%.

The 1970s saw a decline in activity on the health care front. Congress couldn't agree on how to expand health care services, primarily because the economy was in shambles. Any child of the '70s, like me, remembers the long lines for gasoline, chaos in the Middle East, and a fear of nuclear annihilation. We had a lot on our minds . . . although a lot of what we thought about then is sounding eerily familiar today.

Things picked up in the 1980s. Numerous legislative acts expanded coverage to more Americans through Medicaid and Medicare. In 1981, federal law required states to start paying hospitals that provided a disproportionate share of care to Medicaid and uninsured patients (DSH payments). In 1986, Congress passed the Emergency Medical Treatment and Labor Act (EMTALA), which required hospitals to provide service to patients who arrived in the emergency room. As discussed in the Introduction, this law has had a profound effect on the American health care system.

PRICES GET A FRAMEWORK FOR THE FIRST TIME

Arguably, one of the most consequential acts of the 1980s was when Medicare released its Diagnostic Related Groups, or DRGs, in 1983. This was the first time the government established a framework for, ostensibly, a national price list for services. DRGs are codes assigned to procedures performed in a hospital. Today there are about 500 groupings. A commonly used code is DRG 193 for simple pneumonia. There are other DRGs for pneumonia, depending on the severity of the case and other associated complications. The coding system outlines the clinical parameters associated with each DRG.

DRGs enabled Medicare to assign payments to hospitals for each of the conditions identified in each of the codes. Medicare makes a variety of adjustments to these payments based on the types of patients the hospital sees, the cost of the local labor market, and other factors, but the basic framework for payment goes back to the medical care provided for each of the DRG designations.

DRGs opened the door for other coding classifications systems to be incorporated, like Current Procedural Terminology, or CPTs, which were introduced by the American Medical Association (AMA) in 1966.

The DRG classification system has been impactful for two major reasons.

First, coding enabled the automation of the billing processes associated with health care delivery. Electronic records could use DRGs (and other coding structures) as a universally accepted data framework for provider systems. The data collected in these systems gave (and still gives) providers terrific information about their financial and operational performance.

More importantly, DRGs also established Medicare's dominance as the pricing touchstone in the health care industry. Providers and insurers alike began using the codes established by Medicare to create their own price lists and charge masters. Any rates that were set could always be compared to the regularly published Medicare rates. As the years have passed, insurers have become more reliant on Medicare's rates as a means to establish their own. In many cases today, insurers will simply use a markup of Medicare's base rates for their own reimbursement tables.

As a result, much of the pricing in the health care industry today is based less on what a procedure or test or drug actually costs, and more on what the government is willing to pay. Medicare asks hospitals and providers to provide cost data to CMS to help determine local rates for reimbursement and other factors that can influence what they should be paid.

Yet these cost reports are but one input into the complex reimbursement strategy that CMS uses each year. CMS has been increasingly using incentive programs and penalties to impact payments to providers. Providers may get reimbursed at Medicare rates for specific care, but portions of reimbursement categories could be penalized if providers don't achieve targets established by CMS. As noted earlier, hospitals can be penalized for quality issues, for readmitting certain patients, or for higher than allowable mortality rates.

THE LAWS KEPT COMING

Step on up to the '90s, which are marked in memory by the plan that never got passed—the Health Security Act, colloquially known as the Clinton Health Plan.[11] The ambitious plan sought to dramatically reform health care with a blend of regulation and private sector alliances, with all Americans gaining access to some set of health care benefits. Unfortunately, Congress couldn't hammer out the details of how to implement most of the ideas, so the plan never gained any traction.

A notable expansion of insurance coverage during this period was the Children's Health Insurance Program (CHIP), which provides coverage for children whose parents make too much money to qualify for Medicaid. That was signed into law in 1997 and has bipartisan support today.

Congress learned its lesson. For the next fifteen years, radical overhauls to the health care system were abandoned in favor of smaller legislative efforts. What's notable is not the specifics of the laws that were passed, but the fact that the laws just kept coming. Both the Bill Clinton and George W. Bush presidencies were responsible for creating consumer protections and for expanding the scope of government services in health care. Numerous expansions to Medicaid funding were passed, and funding for community health clinics was established.

The granddaddy of data security regulations, the Health Insurance

Portability and Accountability Act (HIPAA), was passed in 1996. One of HIPAA's key features was to establish some guidelines related to protecting health data. It's also one of the reasons why we have to sign extra forms that we never read at the doctor's office so that our doctor can share our medical information with other parties. As will be discussed, data security in the health care industry is a significant issue. We should expect to see more regulations enacted related to protecting patient information.

One of the most notable pieces of legislation passed during this period was the Medicare Prescription Drug, Improvement, and Modernization Act of 2003. It created Medicare Part D, which offers prescription drug coverage for Medicare beneficiaries. The program is popular with seniors, but costs have been growing for several reasons. New drugs, like those introduced in 2013 to cure hepatitis C, have driven up expenses. The use of generic drugs, which are generally cheaper than brand-name drugs, is not leveraged to the degree it could be.

In fact, the secretary of the Department of Health and Human Services (which is over CMS, which runs Medicare) is legally prohibited from negotiating directly with pharmaceutical companies for the prices of Medicare Part D drugs.[12] Medicare is responsible for almost 30% of retail pharmaceutical spending. That means that the pricing for a big chunk of the spending on retail drugs is set by the companies who *make* the drugs. I wish I were making this up, but I'm not.

Then came 2010. President Obama won an overwhelming victory in the presidential race in 2008 and took the momentum as a mandate to enact his campaign slogan—*CHANGE*. The Affordable Care Act was signed into law, millions of previously uninsured Americans got health coverage, and billions of dollars were spent doing it.

The ACA has been the subject of two Supreme Court battles, plenty of failed Republican-led efforts to repeal it, and millions of hours of bickering between leaders at all levels of government. As I've noted previously, the Trump administration has neutered it by overseeing a congressional effort to repeal the individual mandate and by threatening to restrict the government subsidies paid to insurers to reduce the cost of premiums for the majority of individuals who purchase marketplace plans. Efforts are underway to try to eliminate the ability of insurers to discriminate against buyers based on preexisting conditions. President Trump may keep his campaign promise of derailing the ACA, but no replacement plan has been provided. What we're left with is an individual market in tatters, selling the expensive plans that Republicans blamed the ACA for creating.

THE LEGACY OF LAWS

Legislators create laws in response to the demands of their constituencies. Most elected officials behave in accordance with the preferences of their respective electorates (or at least I'd like to think they do). In other words, they advocate for the things that their communities support. When we look back at the breadth of over seventy years' worth of health care-related legislation, we, as citizens, have to recognize that we wanted the benefits and protections that our elected officials created.

The problem now is that the cost to fund all these initiatives has gotten out of control. We have to remember that laws are passed based on the information available at the time they were legislated. Lawmakers can't see into the future. And the CBO can only make financial projections based on known information. When the future turns out differently than was expected when laws were passed, then the costs to fund the regulations also turn out to be different—and usually greater—than what was expected.

When Lyndon B. Johnson's government floated the idea of Medicare, the average life expectancy in America was around seventy years.[13] Today, it's almost eighty years. The program wasn't budgeted for people to live as long as they do, and that's one reason why the federal government spends more than it collects.

The same problem applies to Medicare Part D. As noted, costs in the program grew when new drugs were introduced. George W. Bush's administration didn't see that coming. Nor could it have predicted the explosive growth in research related to precision medicine.

This is a field where drugs are matched to an individual's genetic profile to treat targeted diseases like cancer. These drugs won't be cheap, and Americans will expect that Medicare will figure out a way to pay for (at least some or part of) them.

The cost of the legacy of laws is a stickler for Medicaid too, especially for state governments. As noted, a portion of Medicaid is funded by states. This spending is mandatory and can't be cut by state governments. Most states have some sort of balanced budget amendment, meaning that, in the simplest terms, they can't overspend. As the number of enrollees in the Medicaid program increases, and as provisions for coverage become broader, then the costs to fund Medicaid go up. Assuming the states have a fixed amount of money to spend, they'll have to cut dollars out of other state programs to support things like education and infrastructure, or reduce payouts for pension enrollees.

Despite all the regulations, the government has no overarching strategic approach to health care spending. Today's budgets are driven by yesterday's political battles. Our spending reflects not necessarily what Americans want or need, but on what programs have been agreed upon when circumstances were much different than they are today.

As daunting as it seems, health care regulations are in dire need of a comprehensive review. Politically, it will be a massive legislative challenge. Yet we cannot have financial discipline unless some of the programs are restructured. It won't make anyone happy—but neither will financial Armageddon.

CHAPTER 4

PERSPECTIVES ON HEALTH INSURANCE

In less than a hundred years, health insurance in America has gone from a simple prepaid system to today's administrative megalith. The system's present complications have fueled the nation's passionate demands for better health care, yet no one can agree on exactly what "better health care" truly means.

ACCESS TO HEALTH INSURANCE DOESN'T MAKE PEOPLE HEALTHIER

The historical review of health care reform demonstrates that Americans are looking more and more to the government to provide access to health care services that are affordable for everyone. The government's modus operandi for achieving this goal—be it through Medicaid, Medicare, the Health Security Act, or the Affordable Care

Act—has been to enroll people in an insurance program. Here's the problem: Access to health insurance doesn't make people healthier.

The main purpose of health insurance is to provide individuals with financial security should they incur significant health care expenses. Yet both private and public insurers tout the wellness and prevention features of their programs as a means to keep their members healthy. Clinicians and policy makers appreciate the importance of prevention in maintaining good health. As a result, there's a stubborn belief that individuals with health insurance are more likely to access this preventive care, thereby seeking treatment before health issues can escalate and get out of control.

Yet a good portion of Americans don't use their health insurance to access preventive primary care. In 2015, about 40% of doctor visits were for chronic problems. Another 30% of the visits were for new problems. Only 20% of doctor visits were for preventive care.[1]

Now consider the fact that the key goal of the Affordable Care Act was to expand health care coverage to all Americans. Although the goal was not achieved, the program expanded insurance coverage to over twenty million Americans,[2] and in 2016, the United States notched the lowest rate of uninsured, non-elderly Americans in decades. Yet from the time the ACA was rolled out until today, major health outcome indicators have gotten worse. Longevity has decreased, obesity has increased . . . you know the numbers.

Studies have validated that having health insurance does not necessarily correlate to improved health outcomes, at least when large swaths of the population are viewed in aggregate. An analysis of the impact of RomneyCare, which is the Massachusetts model for universal health care, showed small improvements in the health of residents.[3] A separate, more recent study compared metrics between two states that had expanded coverage through ACA and one that had not.[4] Participants in the expansion states had a 23% bump in "excellent" health. The challenge with tying health improvements to insurance coverage in these studies is that the health improvements were self-reported. Respondents were asked how they felt, meaning the data analyzed was subjective.

Researchers found that expanding Medicaid in Oregon in 2008 increased utilization of services, lowered financial hardships for enrollees, and reduced depression. But key health indicators, like cardiovascular risk, blood pressure, and cholesterol, were not impacted.[5,6]

The Oregon study has been the subject of much academic rebuttal.[7] Subsequent analyses of expanding Medicaid coverage in other states yielded some interesting results. Most notably, mortality rates decreased for those who gained access to health insurance. Such an outcome is positive. However, as will be discussed, mortality rates are affected by a whole host of factors that have nothing to do with health insurance coverage. If having insurance truly improves outcomes, then other key indicators should also show the positive trends akin to the lowered mortality rates.

But they didn't. In fact, the data related to reducing cancer, which is the leading cause of death for individuals aged forty-five to sixty-four,[8] a key age cohort that received expanded coverage, was inconclusive. Having insurance didn't change the metrics related to the disease. It doesn't make sense that mortality rates would go down but the factors contributing to the leading cause of death wouldn't change. Other major health indicators either weren't impacted or weren't studied. The data connecting health insurance to comprehensive positive clinical outcomes just isn't there.

Some have connected the "peace of mind" that health insurance can bring with a better personal outlook on our health. That could be the reason that individuals in these studies felt better, less stressed and less depressed. Americans shouldn't have to worry that an accident or a health condition will leave them financially destitute.

Unfortunately, health care insurance is becoming less effective at providing Americans with the financial security they desire. Premiums and deductibles are on the rise both in the ACA market and for employer-sponsored health plans. Medicare and Medicaid are so taxed that their high spending is threatening the financial security of the country.

Since having health insurance doesn't make the population healthier, and we need to improve the overall health of the American people, we've got to take a hard look at the factors that truly do impact health.

EXTERNAL DETERMINANTS OF HEALTH

A recent, nationwide, decades-long study of Americans showed that insurance status had very little to do with life expectancy. In fact, only 27% of the disparities in different levels of life expectancies among cohorts throughout the country could be attributed to health care factors like having health insurance.[9] Put another way, between 70% and 80% of the reasons individuals die had nothing to do with whether or not they had health insurance coverage. Instead, a variety of socioeconomic and behavioral factors called external determinants to health are the key influencers of health outcomes. Some of these factors include—[10, 11, 12]

- **Genetics**—predisposition to certain diseases, physical attributes, general heartiness
- **Education**—how far your academic career has advanced (which relates to job opportunities), skills to navigate the health care system, and care for yourself
- **Economic Stability**—whether you have a job; savings; can afford housing, food, and other basic human needs
- **Community**—connectedness to community for mental and physical health, access to resources available to feel connected with neighbors
- **Environment**—how safe your home is, concentration of parks and green space, cleanliness of water
- **Food**—having access to enough of the right kinds of food, understanding nutrition
- **Values**—how the belief system of an individual's cultural milieu impacts healthy or unhealthy behaviors (i.e., Southern diets are rich in fatty foods, some communities are known to be very active)
- **Behavior**—controllable factors such as smoking, drinking alcohol, physical exercise

Policy makers, activists, and academicians have long been aware of the role that external determinants play on the health care outcomes. Let's consider education. Studies routinely demonstrate that lower levels of education correlate to poorer health outcomes. Low levels of education impede the development of critical skills like written and verbal communication and reasoning. Some folks may be computer illiterate, which limits their access to basic information and their ability to engage with many constituents in the health care system. For example, they'd need help signing up for insurance coverage on healthcare.gov or other websites. Further, they'd miss out on using important innovations like telemedicine. Given how complicated the health care system is, anyone without a solid educational foundation is at a distinct disadvantage.

Additionally, higher levels of education bring opportunities for better jobs with better pay. That means that individuals with lower levels of education are more likely to be challenged economically. The ripple effect of a low level of education can manifest in an inability to pay for housing in a safe neighborhood. There may not be enough money to buy healthy food, and if there is, there may not be a market within the community that provides it.

As compelling as these externalities are on the lives of individuals and their health outcomes, we can't rely on fixing them as a means to fix our health care system. Blaming the educational system for poor health outcomes implies that fixing it is necessary for health outcomes to improve. We can't wait for that. Nor can we wait for America's income inequality problem to be solved. *Instead, we must acknowledge the relative power of these factors so we can modify our behavior to minimize their impact on our health.*

Consider the following chart. It demonstrates the relative level of control that an individual has on the factors that affect their health.

CHART 8. INDIVIDUAL CONTROL OVER EXTERNAL
DETERMINANTS OF HEALTH

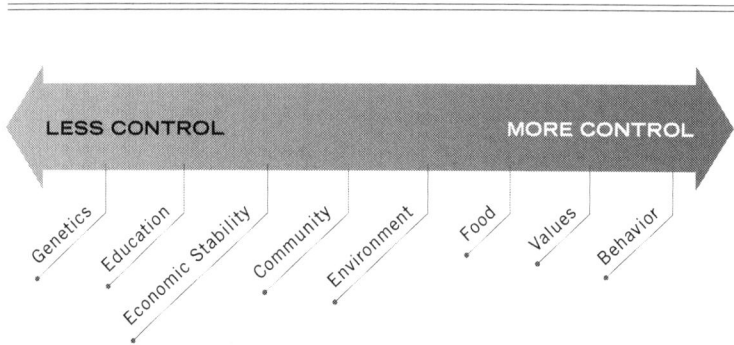

Let's talk genetics. We can't control whether we're born with cerebral palsy or if we'll develop psoriasis in middle age or Parkinson's when we're old. Yet if we could learn more about our genetic predispositions, it would enable us to take steps to minimize or maybe even prevent the onset of specific diseases and conditions. For example, individuals with asthma should avoid living in environments that will exacerbate symptoms, such as those with high pollution or high levels of allergens in the air (like pollen or mold). If genetic information tells us we are predisposed to developing heart disease, we should incorporate cardiac fitness into our lifestyle and monitor the type of foods we eat. If there is a history or a proclivity toward depression and anxiety in our family history, we should proactively seek out a community where deep, trusted bonds can be formed and fostered.

Shifting farther to the right on the chart toward more controllable determinants, individuals may wish to focus on the food they eat. Diets should be modified not only to help avoid the development of genetically influenced conditions but also to optimize health. For example, high levels of salt in a diet can increase your risk of developing hypertension.[13] Upticks in the odds of developing cancer have been connected to the consumption of processed foods.[14] Acknowledging the impact of these types of foods can be beneficial for all of us.

One of the more challenging but controllable externalities relates to American values and cultural norms about health. Our country glorifies athletes, yet the average American is overweight. There's an abundance of programming about food preparation—there's an entire television network devoted to it—yet fewer and fewer of us take the time to cook for ourselves. Instead of enjoying the organic and healthy food options that have made a significant impact on our grocery shelves, we eat more salt and preservative-laden prepackaged and restaurant food.

It's obvious that we can't expect the health care system to correct the problems that are generated by cultural norms or social and economic inequities in different aspects of our nation. Even health plans loaded with benefits and generous financial coverage can't address the root causes of poor health. *We need to dial back the expectation of what the health care system is supposed to do, and think more about what we can do.*

SPENDING WHAT WE SHOULD, NOT WHAT WE CAN

For starters, we can support a governmental approach to health care spending that is more disciplined and controlled. Budgeting should not be based on how much we *could* spend on health care but on how much we *should* spend.

America is a nation that espouses the notion of equality and fairness. Our cultural association with equality is rooted in the Declaration of Independence. The words "We hold these truths to be self-evident, that all men are created equal . . . " are an essential part of what it means to be an American. All Americans, regardless of gender, race, economic status, religious affiliation, and sexual orientation have an equal opportunity to pursue the American Dream.

Yet when it comes to health, we are far from equal. In fact, no equality exists in our health status because each of us comes into the world with a certain health makeup. Some of us have a genetic predisposition to colon cancer. Others have a history of heart disease. And some of us are born with birth defects. There's nothing equal or fair about being born with spina bifida.

If we are trying to level the health playing field from a budgeting perspective, equality in health care should mean that everyone should be provided with the same access and the same amount of resources for each of their health care needs. But this postulation is problematic because some people require more support than others based on their health status at birth; they simply need more access, which makes them more expensive individuals to treat. How do we fairly allocate resources when everyone's predisposed needs for health care are different?

Further, external determinants of health feature heavily into an individual's health status. The health problems that one person has may be the result of factors totally out of their control (like genetics). Someone else's poor health status could be the result of behaviors completely within their control (like excessive drinking and drug use). A policy maker can't decipher the difference, and in the case of children, what's the solution? We can't punish obese children when their parents are responsible for their health and well-being.

Americans also believe in individual freedom. That's why it's legal for pregnant women (of a designated age) to smoke and drink alcohol. It's also legal for the rest of us to smoke and drink, even though the detrimental aspects of these behaviors are well documented.

We can't clamp down on individual freedom. We can't determine who's behaving badly on purpose and who's just the victim of bad luck (or some combination thereof). So the present health care system in America has evolved into one that satisfies the lowest common denominator. Everyone is entitled to the health care they need no matter how, who, or why they are like they are.

Today's system uses some clinical guidelines, regulatory requirements, and the opinion of physicians and caregivers to approve access to care. The language included in health plans and regulations requires that what is deemed medically necessary by a physician must oftentimes be covered by an insurer. ACA regulations have forbidden insurers from issuing lifetime caps on how much they must spend on an individual enrolled in their plan. Nor can they cap annual spending (meaning the care they must fund) per person. Such an approach is consumer friendly—and fiscally dangerous.

This problem is exacerbated by the fact that the cost to treat certain health conditions is becoming increasingly dependent on the pharmaceutical and surgical options that are available. What this means is that a disease that can be cured with drugs or surgery will end up being more expensive to treat than a disease that has few to no medical options available. Consider an individual who is born blind. From a payment perspective, it is a relatively inexpensive condition to treat since there is no cure for blindness. (There are social services for the blind that are funded through Medicaid. But the majority of these costs are not related to direct medical care, like drugs and surgeries, that are used extensively to treat other conditions.)

Now consider an individual with Crohn's disease, a chronic condition affecting the lining of the digestive tract. There is no cure for Crohn's either. Yet over the last decade, a raft of new therapies has come to market to treat its symptoms, and doctors must use trial and error to determine which type of approach will work most effectively for different patients.[15] The health care system could spend very little (for good old-fashioned antibiotics) or upward of hundreds of thousands of dollars (for surgery or sophisticated biologics[16]) on treatment methods.

The Crohn's example echoes the earlier discussion about how new treatments can burden the system with costs simply because they weren't previously available. It also identifies a budgeting problem associated with clinical variability. Some doctors may be high spenders, trying the most expensive treatments first. If those treatments fail, they move on to the next and the next, spending money all along the way. Others may be better diagnosticians who can match treatment options effectively to what specific patients need. Since the health care system can't know which treatments will work best for which patients, it must rely on the judgment of physicians. That creates significant variability in spending.

SOMETHING'S GOT TO GIVE

We spend billions of dollars on health insurance, yet our outcomes are getting worse and worse. We look to health insurance to make us well when most of the factors impacting our health have nothing to do with it. Each medical innovation increases the amount of money that could be spent on health care, pushing spending to uncontrollable levels. The current model of health insurance simply doesn't work. We need new ideas that provide fair access to care that also ensures fiscal responsibility.

CHAPTER 5

ATTEMPTS AT HEALTH CARE TRANSFORMATION

Everyone from politicians to academicians, clinicians, administrators, entrepreneurs, investors, and regular Joes and Janes wants to find a way to make the American health system run better. We've all got a vested interest in it. Tens of billions of dollars have been invested in technologies and programs that are supposed to transform the industry. Countless hours of political wrangling and legislative effort have expended. Article after article has been written about it. Yet despite the development of new solutions and ideas, health care seems to get more complicated and costlier. Why hasn't anyone been able to crack the code?

Three transformative concepts that have been considered ground breaking solutions to our health care challenges will be discussed in this and the following chapters:

1. Electronic medical records

2. Single payer system

3. Value-based care

Each of these ideas has considerable merit, and they have all been projected to radically transform the industry. Unfortunately, none of them have, and none of them will. I will explain why these opportunities failed (or will fail) to satisfy expectations. This discussion will provide an in-depth understanding of the industry's complexities and set the stage for why the Dream Plan would be an effective alternative to our current system.

ELECTRONIC MEDICAL RECORDS

Electronic medical records (EMRs) store medical and demographic information about patients in an electronic format. It is arguably the most hyped technology to ever hit the health care industry. EMRs were supposed to save the industry half a trillion dollars over a fifteen-year period ending in 2017.[1] Such a platform was expected to give practitioners quick and easy access to patient information. Gone would be the need to track down paper records in different parts of the hospital or from different locations to provide clinicians with the information they need to provide accurate and timely treatment. Operationally, EMRs were expected to be a godsend.

But the real benefits were supposed to come from the enhancements to patient outcomes. Physicians would be able to access a comprehensive medical history during both routine visits and emergency episodes. For example, doctors would have access to prescription history as well as any drug allergies, which could prevent adverse reactions to medications that might be used in an emergency. They would know whether a woman is pregnant, and that information could impact a clinical protocol that could save her life and that of her baby, regardless of what stage of pregnancy she is in.

Further, it was hoped that data from multiple records could be viewed in aggregate across a community, county, or state—even across the country. This perspective, called population health management, was intended to provide insights into regional health patterns, identify barriers to better outcomes, and even offer opportunities for the development of new drugs, goods, and services. EMRs were supposed to save the industry billions of dollars while transforming the delivery of care.

Today, almost all hospitals have implemented some version of an EMR. They've spent billions of dollars doing it, but the transformational aspects of the technology have yet to be realized. There are several factors playing into these lackluster results.

First off, we can always blame the government, given its tendency to see a good idea and regulate the hell out of it. The feds, like everyone else, saw the potential of an EMR-connected country. Beginning with the Health Information Technology for Economic and Clinical Health (HITECH) Act in 2009, providers were required to implement technology that collected a designated set of information in a somewhat shareable format. Millions of dollars were set aside to promote and reward adaption, and penalties were put in place for the failure to do so.

It's important to note that many hospitals were already using EMRs before this legislation went into effect. The HITECH Act pushed the remaining holdouts into the EMR space, but it also encouraged many providers to replace their current technology. The legislation sought to establish data standards called "meaningful use," and some of the legacy systems didn't comply with the regs. Further, cloud-based solutions that are nimbler and theoretically easier to install came on the market. This enticed providers to go whole-hog into a technological transformation of their operations.

While the feds pushed providers to adapt the technology, implementing it successfully was another story altogether. Anyone who's worked in information technology (IT) knows the challenges related to implementation. One of the most epic fails in health care technology history was the botched rollout of the healthcare.gov website[2] in 2013. Like many IT projects, its costs were way over budget, and then it crashed—for days—after it was launched.

Implementing EMRs are expensive, too. Partners HealthCare in

Boston, one of the nation's leading health systems, spent over a billion dollars implementing EMR powerhouse Epic. Now they're tasked with the costs of maintaining it, which can run millions of dollars a year. That's just one system. There are over 5,500 hospitals in America . . . you do the math.

Further, EMRs were supposed to make the physician's job easier. But using one requires a whole lot of data entry. In fact, physicians reportedly spend more than half their day on data-entry activities.[3] They spend more and more time inputting information into an EMR and less and less time on patient-facing activities. Such a shift in provider focus decreases the quality of care, which is the opposite intent of the implementation of the EMR. Sadly, being forced to spend so much time on data entry has become a major factor in physician burnout and dissatisfaction.

INTEROPERABILITY

The HITECH Act wasn't just about getting EMRs installed; it was also about the promotion of interoperability, or the creation of common formats by which different providers could share information. This is the aspect of the legislation that has gotten the least traction but is necessary for the EMRs to achieve many of their sought-after goals. How can a complete patient history be reviewed if data in one system isn't accessible from another? How can comprehensive health trends be evaluated if only certain pieces of data from certain sources for certain patients can be analyzed?

Industry-wide interoperability has been hampered by a variety of factors, and first among them is the concern about data security. The American health care system, aside from being expensive, inefficient, and sometimes ineffective, has another ominous claim to fame: Most Hacked Industry.[4] Data breaches are commonplace in hospitals and other provider networks.

Contrary to what you might think, hackers aren't blazing through firewalls to learn whether or not you've got an STD. They want access to the comprehensive demographic and historical information contained in health records that can enable them to gain access to your financial records, learn about your family, steal your identity, and foment fraudulent claims.

Of course, both patients and providers are very concerned about data security. Consider a fifty-something, unemployed professional who's got early-stage Parkinson's. That's not something he wants on a job application. And some hackers may very well use juicy personal tidbits about your health status to extort you or the ones close to you.

Providers have a legal responsibility to keep your personal health information (PHI) safe. They face financial penalties when certain security breaches occur. The last thing they want is a lawsuit. As a result, providers are incented to hold and protect the data, not to share it.

Now consider interoperability from the perspective of the EMR company. Making connections between IT systems requires cooperation, which means that competing organizations have to work together. Companies may have to share proprietary information about their products, like how their databases are constructed or how their security is configured. Even if data is pulled from a number of systems into a neutral database, there's still a problem. Simply knowing what information is stored and how easily it can be shared could give away privileged information about a company's products.

Unfortunately, the biggest problem in achieving interoperability in health care is that there is no financial incentive for any single constituent to do it. The government, hospitals, and insurers all have a stake in supporting interoperability, but the biggest beneficiary of sharing health data is the patient. Finding a way to provide a service that coordinates the collection, storage, and shareability of a patient's health data in a secure manner at an affordable price is hard to fathom, given how our system is set up.

But don't tell that to Apple. They are leading the charge in their attempts to develop a personal EMR. Their health app allows patients to store selected PHI that is uploaded by participating providers.[5] This allows the patient to share data across multiple locations. It's a great start to promoting data sharing, and right now it's free. How long do you think that's going to last?

On a more optimistic note, we should be grateful for the inroads that Apple is making in their attempts to create interoperability. At least they have recognized that the data should reside with the patient, because the patient is the one constant point of contact in every health care delivery transaction. Maybe the next generation of Americans will have the ultimate in a portable EMR: an implanted microchip that stores all their data for every single transaction right under their skin.

CHAPTER 6

THE CASE AGAINST A SINGLE PAYER SYSTEM

Many Americans believe that the answer to our health care ills lies in the centralization of health care services into a single payer system run by the government. Access to care would be more democratic since everyone would be on the same insurance plan. The costs associated with contracting and paying multiple vendors would be reduced, because there would only be one source of funds. Further, the health records of every American would be centralized, enabling the government to use this data to better manage patient populations around the country.

Over the past few years, interest in a single payer system in America has gained traction. Gallup estimates that almost half of Americans want a government-run health system, the largest percentage tracked by the organization since it started polling Americans on the topic in 2010.[1] The issue was a favorite of progressives during the 2016 presidential election. Democratic candidate Bernie Sanders's "Medicare for All" proposal was a rallying point for many of his supporters. It has become a much-discussed potential platform issue for the national Democratic Party.

Many other industrialized nations use a single payer system with relative success, which seems to serve as proof of the model's potential effectiveness for America. As noted in the following chart, these other countries spend less per capita on health care than we do in America.[2]

CHART 9. 2016 HEALTH CARE COSTS PER CAPITA
BY HIGH INCOME NATIONS

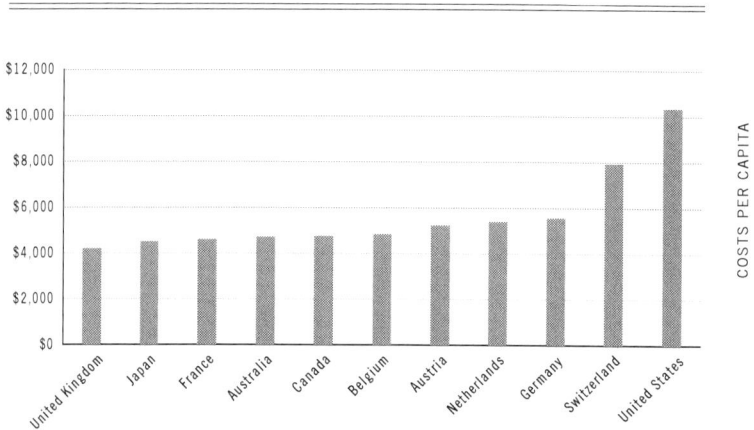

The United States spent $10,348 per capita on health care in 2016. This figure is almost 31% larger than Switzerland's per capita spending, which is the second highest in the comparison study.

As far as outcomes, we trail comparator nations in many critical categories. Our mortality rates are higher than everyone else's. More patients are admitted to hospitals for preventable conditions, like congestive heart failure and diabetes. And the American health care system is responsible for more medical errors in certain areas than are tracked in other countries.[3]

While many of these comparator nations do a far better job with costs and outcomes, most of their health care systems are not sole, single payer systems. Some citizens in most of these countries buy supplemental insurance from private companies. The models are more akin to the American Medicare model, where a set of services are covered by the government, and then individuals can opt to buy health insurance to augment their coverage. This is the model in the United Kingdom, Germany, Australia, and Japan.

Comparing costs and selected performance metrics of the American health care system to that of other industrialized nations is but one aspect of study that can help us determine if a single payer is right for America. There are distinctions about America's size, culture, and composition that also require serious consideration.

SIZE

While many European countries are first-world nations like America, the size of our populations is seismically dissimilar. Germany is the most populous nation in Europe with a population of over eighty-two million (assuming we exclude the Russian Federation and Turkey, both of which straddle Europe and Asia). That's about a quarter the size of the United States. The size of other European nations trails off from there. More people live in New York City than do in the entire country of Switzerland. Switzerland's population is comparable to Virginia's, with a little over eight million people.

We can all comprehend the idea that managing something small is easier than managing something large. But sometimes bringing smaller entities together can be beneficial. In the business world, one reason that companies consolidate is to take advantage of economies of scale. The more units—be it people, products, terabytes—that can be managed under an efficient infrastructure, the lower the per-unit cost of operating the business. More favorable deals can be cut with combined negotiating power and competitive positions are improved when companies join forces.

All of this works as long as the infrastructure doesn't get bloated and too bureaucratic. When it does, the organization reaches a state of diseconomies of scale. More costs are added to manage the system, but the system can't generate any more savings. At this point, the unit costs start to go up, not down.

In fact, the size of government in America is three and a half times larger today than it was fifty-five years ago.[4] One estimate claims that the activities and the associated economic impact of complying with regulations costs the American economy $1.9 trillion a year.[5] Given health care's outsized role in our country, the scale of the bureaucracy is becoming problematic for the industry.

We've already discussed the myriad laws that have been passed related to health care policy. The ACA itself was at about a thousand pages of legislation,[6] although other counts, which factor in proposed rules and notices related to the legislation and retyping it to a more readable format, peg it at tens of thousands of pages.[7] CMS and other regulatory bodies demand so much reporting that the American Hospital Association estimates that the cost to comply with regulations for every patient admitted to a hospital is $1,200.[8] When it comes to America's regulatory environment, we have reached the point of diseconomies of scale.

The simplest argument against the single payer system is the overspending in the public health programs. As has been discussed at length in this book, costs associated with the Medicare program are wreaking havoc on our economic underpinnings. The costs for Medicaid are significantly impacting state budgets, too. If we can't keep these programs under control at their current size, why does anyone think that expanding them won't make things exponentially worse?

We need the government to support efforts to ensure patient safety and quality. But there is a difference between the government's role in establishing effective and well-crafted rules and using the power of its magnitude to run the entire thing.

CULTURE AND COMPOSITION

While many like to point to the strong performance of health care systems in Europe, one country trumps them all in terms of outcomes: Japan. Of nations with over a million inhabitants, Japan has the longest life expectancy in the world and the lowest mortality rates for neonatal births (meaning that premature babies have the best chance of survival in Japan). It ranks fifth in the world for mortality rates for children under five years old.[9] The list goes on. The Japanese have health care figured out.

Much of the country's strong health outcomes relate to a cultural phenomenon absent in the United States and present in many of the European countries with single payer systems: ethnic homogeneity. Japan's population is 98.5% Japanese,[10] making it one of the least diverse countries in the world.

Managing the health needs of a homogeneous population is easier than managing a diverse one because there's one set of behaviors, values, and cultural practices to evaluate. Of course, with about 130 million people in Japan, there are many subsets of the population with culturally distinctive practices. But by and large, the diet, the work ethic, and the behaviors of the population at a macro level are similar. That makes the development of a national health care system much more efficient because the health care needs of only one type of individual must be accommodated.

One of America's most significant assets, our diversity, makes it hard for a single payer system to function well in our country. According to the U.S. Census Bureau, the largest ethnic group in America is whites, at 60.7%.[11] The opioid epidemic is impacting the white population much more than the African American or Hispanic communities.[12] Hispanic Americans represent 18.1% of the population. The leading cause of death in America is cardiovascular disease. But for Hispanics, it's cancer.[13] African Americans, who represent 13.4% of the population, are disproportionately affected by diabetes.[14] In order for the health care system to be effective, the government must address the varying health issues impacting the myriad constituencies in the country. It's no easy task.

The United States isn't only ethnically diverse. We're geographically diverse. Our country sits in five different time zones and ranges from the tropical (Hawaii) to the frigid (Alaska). We have mountain ranges, deserts, plains, coastal communities. Each of these areas has different climates, food sources, and behaviors. Massachusetts is considered the healthiest state in America,[15] and the military has trouble finding fit recruits in the South.[16] Coastal states enjoy seafood, and landlocked states celebrate red meat. In a single payer system, the government would be significantly challenged to drive down costs through preventive, targeted care because the communities across America are so diverse.

A health system must respond to these differences with tailored action plans. Differences require customization. Customization kills efficient regulation.

FRAUD

When taking the Hippocratic Oath, physicians commit to perform their craft with professional integrity and ethical standards. Unfortunately, not everyone lives by these noble standards, and some providers bilk the system out of money. The temptation to do so is appealing because the complexity of the Medicare and Medicaid programs make them highly susceptible to fraud.

The Government Accountability Office (GAO) investigates and reports on all types of government spending, including funds allocated to health care. It has considered Medicare an "at-risk" program for improper spending since 1990.[17] In fiscal 2014, 48% of all the federal government's improper payments were associated with the Medicare program.[18] Another 14% were associated with Medicaid. That year, about 10% of Medicare's entire payments were fraudulent, accounting for about $60 billion in improper payments. Digging deeper, the error rates associated with specific Medicare programs like DME (durable medical equipment) and Home Health were over 50%.

Improper payments in Medicare are so rampant that there's

actually a task force devoted to addressing the problem. It's called the Medicare Fraud Strike Force. (Is there an opportunity for a new movie franchise here? I hope not.) The organization began in 2007, and as of January 2018, it was responsible for identifying over 1,938 criminal actions associated with over $3 billion in fraud.[19] As impressive as that may seem, the figure has to be put in context. As noted, in 2014, Medicare was defrauded by close to $60 billion.

Adding to the size and scope of government programs by expanding coverage to all Americans will add to potential losses due to fraudulent behavior.

CHOICE

The American consumer-based culture demands choice. We are a nation that consumes eleven different types of M & M candies[20]—and that excludes the holiday versions. There are sixteen types of Cheerios[21] on grocery store aisles (usually across from the candy, which is a savvy move vis-à-vis product placement and an interesting commentary about how Americans shop for food).

Technology has enabled many of us not to need to go to the grocery store anymore. We can order up a personal grocery shopper, have food delivered, or have meal kits placed on our doorstep. There's a prepared food option available in almost every retail outlet from convenience stores to department stores to drugstores. We can eat in a restaurant, eat in our car, assemble food in a shop and take it home, and even, yes, cook for ourselves.

Now think about all the different kinds of ways that we can shop for clothes.

Or find transportation.

Or buy a house.

Americans demand options. There's no way Americans would tolerate one choice for health care. It's simply not in our cultural DNA.

CONCLUSION

As a final point, many conservatives, and that includes an opinion held by Ronald Reagan, oppose a single payer system because they contend that it subsidizes care for the rich. Some object to Medicare because tax dollars committed to the program wind up paying for the health care of individuals who can afford to pay for it themselves.

This argument fails the logic test for two reasons. First, many believe the intent of a single payer system is to make health care more democratic. Forcing the rich into a system that everyone else has to use makes sure that every American has similar access to care.

The second and more relevant point is that the rich pay the vast majority of the taxes. Think about it: the richest 20% of Americans pay 87% of income taxes.[22] The rich aren't getting their care subsidized, they're paying for it—and for almost everyone else's, too.

There are plenty of reasons to object to a single payer solution. Given the complexities in the health care system, we need to scale back on the role of government, not ramp it up. What needs to be considered is the amount of waste that is generated by paying the government to oversee the health care system versus just using the money to pay for care directly. That would be a different kind of single payer system—where the single payer is you.

CHAPTER 7

VALUE-BASED CARE: AN ACADEMIC POLICY SOLUTION

Value-based care (VBC) is a concept born from academic circles, embraced by policy makers, and cautiously accepted by providers. It's a simple idea—one that requires providers to be paid based on the value that they deliver to patients. The concept has slowly worked its way into the health care payment system, but as of now, there's much more hype than proven results.

In the early 2000s, the seminal book *Redefining Health Care: Creating Value-Based Competition on Result*s by Michael Porter and Elizabeth Teisberg was released. The book proposes a way to apply the competitive forces that shape other industries to the dysfunctional health care system. *Redefining Health Care* and the subsequent articles, seminars, and classes have made value-based care the most influential academic concept to impact health care in our generation.

The challenge, of course, is to see if such an approach to paying for care could work in practical application. In order for that to happen, our current approach to paying for health care, the fee-for-service (FFS) model, would have to change.

AMERICA'S CURRENT FFS PAYMENT SYSTEM

In the FFS model, providers are paid based on the number of visits, tests, and surgeries performed. Providers are incented to do as many transactions as possible to maximize their pay. Such behavior can drive up utilization without an associated improvement in health.

America's high utilization problem is well documented. Compared to other high-income nations, our health care system uses the highest volume of diagnostic imaging.[1] The average American takes between two to three pills a day, which is higher than other countries. Increasingly, studies are indicating that aggressive surgeries for diseases such as prostate or breast cancer may be performed at unnecessarily high rates. In other words, some patients may be advised to undergo a radical mastectomy despite the fact that the procedure may not affect the patient's mortality.

Further, the concentration of health care that an individual utilizes accelerates toward the end of life. This shouldn't be a surprise, given that there are increasingly voluminous ways to keep a person alive and, therefore, for a provider to be paid. This does not mean that all doctors are motivated to maximize their own financial gain, but there are inconsistencies in care. A variety of treatments may be performed on one patient, while a patient with a similar health profile might achieve the same health outcome despite receiving little to no care.[2]

One rationale for the high-volume approach to medicine is that some providers overtest as a defensive maneuver to protect themselves from potential legal action. Right now, there is no federal limit on medical malpractice claims. That brings attorneys into the mix, many of whom engage in aggressive lawsuits against physicians, hospitals, and corporations. While discussions to cap these awards are underway,[3] we have an overly litigious society. Ironically, many doctors behave in ways that may seem financially motivated because they have to guard against attorneys who are also behaving in ways that may be financially motivated.

In any case, something needed to be done to address the overutilization issue. As part of the ACA, several initiatives, including the Bundled Payments for Care Improvement (BPCI) initiative,[4] were funded to explore ways for providers to embrace VBC. A stash of cash was set aside to be given to different providers if they were able to come up with ways to create VBC models for different clinical conditions.

In other words, the government had no distinct plan about how to implement VBC. They had to pay the providers to try to figure it out.

Years later, VBC has come a long way from the lofty aspirations of a value-focused system envisaged in *Redesigning Health Care*. It has become, for all intents and purposes, a cost-cutting tool more appropriately referred to as bundled payments.

Both public and private payers are creating bundles of services for a designated activity, and they're paying providers one flat fee for the care. This bundled approach is great for payers because it's basically a form of a volume discount. They group services together and pay less for the bundle than they would if they paid separately for each activity.

One area where bundled payments are starting to gain traction is in the ambulatory surgery center (ASC) environment. There are three bills associated with surgical care provided in an ASC: one for the anesthesiologist, one for the professional fee (i.e., the surgeon), and one for the facility (that covers the actual site of care, the salaries of the nurses, the supplies, etc.). Some commercial payers are lumping all three of those fees together and paying the surgery center a single, lower rate. The provider is likely to agree to this option if the payer proposing the bundle is a significant revenue contributor to the facility. As long as everyone—the anesthesiologist, the physician, and the center—is still making a profit, getting paid a little less is better than getting paid nothing at all.

Pure value-based care should improve outcomes while also lowering costs. The above model might not do much of either. From an outcomes perspective, the cases performed in an outpatient environment are not exactly ripe for dramatic improvements. The types of procedures that are performed in this setting are not as complicated as those done in a hospital. Patients must be medically approved to receive their care in an outpatient setting. As a result, outcomes in the outpatient environment are much more predictable. Improving the value delivered will be incremental because the subset of patients under evaluation are, by definition, already expected to have positive outcomes.

Costs certainly are reduced for the payer because they pay less overall for the same set of services. Yet the administrative costs for the provider increase. When the payer only has to make one payment rather than three, it puts the administrative burden on the provider to collect the appropriate billing information and to distribute the payments. Ordinarily, the three constituencies involved—the anesthesiologist, the surgeon, and the facility—are not using the same technology to process payments. Manual processes, which can cause errors and add time, are often used. As noted earlier, faxing is still a standard mode of communication. So much for innovations in care delivery.

There are more opportunities to improve care and reduce cost on complicated inpatient procedures. These were the target of the ACA legislation. It sought to bundle payments for Medicare patients undergoing certain complex procedures like a coronary artery bypass graft (CABG) commonly performed during open-heart surgery. Given that heart disease is the number one killer in America, there's an incredible opportunity for savings by reforming some of the clinical activities related to treating it. From a business case perspective, it makes a lot of sense to apply VBC to this type of procedure.

Yet the practical realities of applying VBC to complex cases like CABG have proven to be overwhelming. No doubt there is a basic set of costs and activities that are associated with the procedure. A VBC payment model can identify costs for the basic set of services and set a reimbursement rate. That rate is likely to be lower than the sum of all the parts, which lowers costs for the payer, Medicare.

But there can be considerable variability in the actual delivery of care based on a whole host of factors, including the patient's age, weight, and co-morbidities (meaning whether they have other diseases like diabetes or hypertension that can make the procedure more challenging). Adjustment factors can be used to try to modify the base reimbursement figure to account for these factors. But with so many calculations, the ability to accurately reimburse a provider for the care can get complicated.

In addition, providers have the operational challenge of processing value-based payments using existing technology. Today's EMRs have been designed around optimizing payments in the FFS world, one procedure, one visit, one encounter at a time. The systems simply haven't been built to accept a single payment for multiple encounters. Given that hundreds of billions of dollars have been spent implementing EMRs, no one's going to spend more money to replace them. Provider costs will inevitably go up as they must pay the administrative fees associated with processing payments for VBC using their FFS technology.

The real issue comes in identifying what "value" is and in determining who's responsible for achieving the VBC goals. There are two parties in the provider/patient relationship, and it only takes one of them to behave badly for the value-based model to fail.

Consider a patient who requires a knee replacement. The outcome for an eighty-five-year-old grandmother might be her ability to walk without a cane or walk up a flight of stairs. For an NFL wide receiver, he'll need full mobility. His contract and his livelihood depend upon it. No institutionalized system can account for the variances in outcomes that every American might want—or in what would be necessary to achieve them.

Solutions would need to rely on more adjustment factors. Odds are the grandmother's surgery would cost more than the football player's, and that increase may be incorporated in an adjusted rate the provider is reimbursed for the care. But VBC assumes that a portion of the payment will also be tied to the outcome. And that's where the accountability issue makes using a VBC model for payment inefficacious.

The grandmother probably needs more time to recover and will need more physical therapy than the football player. The resources that one would expect to use for these two different situations would vary, and the timetable for recovery would be different. Let's assume the adjustment factors accurately capture these differences in what would be required of these two patients to achieve their respective outcomes.

But what happens if the football player is cut from his team, falls into a depression, and loses all motivation to get better? What if he simply doesn't go to physical therapy and doesn't meet the risk-adjusted time period for recovery? In a case like that, the provider gets penalized, even though the reasons for the poor outcome are completely out of their control.

Providers should be measured on the factors they can control—like medical errors and infection rates. But if a patient doesn't take his medications, or clean his wounds, or get the appropriate rest, he may have an adverse outcome that is the result of his own behavior. The presumption of innocence for the doctor does not exist in the value-based care world. The provider is assumed to be guilty of poor clinical care unless the patient has a good outcome, regardless of how the patient behaves.

It is clear that our fee-for-service model drives up costs and needs to be addressed. But the theory of value-based care as a reimbursement model has yet to be proven in implementation. The Trump administration is decidedly less regulatorily motivated than the Obama administration and has shifted away from some of the bundled payment initiatives.[5] Many believe this is premature and that the VBC models have not had time to evolve.

I think the VBC model is a great idea—as long as the metrics aren't completely regulated by the government, and the prices are established in a consumer-based market. Every single one of us wants to receive the appropriate care necessary to address our health concerns in a respectful, efficient manner. We are all individuals, and our care needs should be tailored to our unique demands. We just need a different payment model to do it.

AMERICA'S
HEALTH CARE SYSTEM

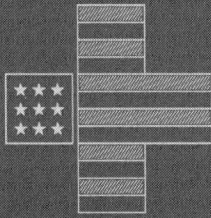

THE DREAM
PLAN

A BLUE SKY PROPOSAL

The Dream Plan is a clean slate, blue sky proposal for a new American health care system, assuming we were to start all over from scratch. In this model, the health care system as we know it today would no longer exist. Medicare, Medicaid, and broad-based health insurance coverage would be replaced with an alternative payment strategy and a modified approach to public health. What we've come to expect from the health care system would completely change.

The Dream Plan assumes that individuals would save money over the course of their lives to pay for their own health care expenses. Those who do not have the means to afford their own care will default into a public health system, funded by taxes and other resources. Everyone would have health coverage in the Dream Plan.

The cornerstone of the Dream Plan is a Longitudinal Health Care Plan (LHCP). The LHCP is a cross between a personal health record and an investment vehicle. It is a new kind of product that could be offered by banks, insurers, or any organization that can provide the services required to help its customers manage their money so they can manage their own health.

The LHCP would have three major components. The first, called a Conditions Timeline, would be a personalized chronology of the diseases and conditions that an individual is likely to develop over the course of his or her lifetime. A Genetic Analysis would create a base profile of potential health conditions for each customer. This information would be complemented by a robust evaluation of the many factors that influence an individual's health, such as their behavior, occupation, income, geography, values, etc.

The second component, the Financial Commitment, attaches the costs to treat and manage all of the conditions identified in the Timeline. These costs, in turn, would be used as the basis to develop an investment plan. Individuals would be advised on how much to save so that they could pay for all of their health care needs independently.

The power of the Dream Plan is that it allows individuals to see the future and then work backward to make their lives healthier and more productive in the present. The third aspect of the LHCP, the Customer Action Report (CAR), is an annually generated report that provides this service. The CAR would be developed with input from both medical professionals and investors. It would provide a number of action-oriented functions including advice about behavioral modifications that could improve health as well as the financial implications of complying with the recommendations. In other words, the CAR could identify health goals, such as weight loss, which could forestall the projected development of a condition, such as heart disease, by several years. That, in turn, could reduce the customer's financial obligation.

Individuals who do not have the resources to fund an LHCP will be covered in the public health program. The Dream Plan's public health solution varies from today's Medicaid program in a number of ways. Today, individuals have to apply to Medicaid and meet certain qualifications. In the Dream Plan, those who could not afford to pay for their care through an LHCP would automatically default into the public health program. Care access for those on public health would be modeled using the care plans developed by average Americans who have an LHCP. This allows for the democratization of health care. Program dollars would be capped based on these budgets. In some cases, staying on budget will require care to be rationed. Basic services would be covered for all, but a distinction would be made for individuals who require access to nonessential services. Those who satisfy work and volunteer requirements, as well as individuals who visit a primary care doctor each year, would be given preferential access to care.

Be it through a public or private program, all Americans would be incented to manage their own health by coordinating closely with a primary care physician. Strengthening the importance of the patient/provider partnership is one of the critical success factors in the Dream Plan. Together, the team would be charged with developing health care protocols that match each patient's value system. Doing so enhances patient engagement, reduces costs, and most importantly, improves health outcomes.

Readers: Meet the Dream Plan.

CHAPTER 8

LONGITUDINAL HEALTH CARE PLAN

The core aspect of the Dream Plan is the creation of a Longitudinal Health Care Plan (LHCP). The LHCP is a personalized account that allows individuals to fund their own health care expenses over the course of their lives. It's a hybrid between a personal health record and an investment fund.

PATIENTS ARE NOW CUSTOMERS

Prior to this point, I have used the word "patient" to refer to an individual when discussing his or her relationship with the health care system. In this section, I will refer to individuals as "customers." I want to present the Dream Plan through the lens of someone who would be contracting with a company that offers an LHCP.

There will be portions of the LHCP experience that are distinctly medical. LHCP customers are also patients when they have their annual physical and when they engage in all their provider-based activities. But I will still refer to the individual as a customer because I will be focusing on how the information that is generated from these interactions will impact the data in the LHCP.

The Dream Plan elevates the importance of the primary care provider in the health care ecosystem because LHCP customers will need to partner with these professionals to develop customized care plans. Medical professionals will be critical in communicating how the data generated by the LHCP should impact a customer's behavior. Trusted, long-term relationships will help ensure follow-through on the protocols outlined in the LHCP.

This book does not specify how the physician will access the data in the LHCP or how data from medical exams will be transferred to the companies operating the LHCP. This data transfer is essential and must be conducted securely. But the mechanics of how it happens— via secure connection between the physician and the LHCP provider, a paper hand off coordinated by the customer, or some other transfer—will be worked out as LHCPs are brought to market.

HOW WE'LL ACCESS LHCPS

LHCPs are a new kind of "product." I will outline the features that could be included in an LHCP, but there will be different versions of how such an offering could manifest when it is actually created. In other words, when a company starts to develop an LHCP, it may focus more on some of the modules described below than others. The company may eliminate some or add new features. LHCPs will be different depending on which company is offering them and based on what customers want.

LHCPs could become products offered by banks. Imagine that J.P. Morgan offers an LHCP. You, the customer, would open an LHCP account with J.P. Morgan, and the functions outlined in this chapter would be coordinated by the financial institution. The bank may partner with health care practitioners or other business providers to conduct some of the features not traditionally performed by a bank, particularly with regard to the activities identified in the Conditions Timeline. But the investment activities would be performed in-house using the bank's expertise in financial services.

Alternatively, insurers could offer LHCPs. Their expertise in health data and their understanding of local markets could give them a competitive advantage over other potential LHCP providers. Insurers might then contract with financial services companies to provide the capabilities for the investment aspect of the product, or they could do it in-house themselves. In fact, hospitals or physician groups may wish to provide LHCPs too. The product could be offered by any organization that has the capabilities to deliver the services required. In the end, customers will determine which products are the most effective based on how the different versions of the LHCP perform over time.

LHCP MODULES

The LHCP is divided into three major sections: the Conditions Timeline, the Financial Commitment, and the Customer Action Report. The Conditions Timeline is the repository for the customer's health information. The Financial Commitment section converts the health information into an investment strategy for the customer. The Customer Action Report outlines steps the LHCP holder can take to improve their health and track their investments.

There are seven modules to the LHCP. The Conditions Timeline and the Financial Commitment each include three modules. The Customer Action Plan is the final module.

CHART 10. SEVEN MODULES OF THE LHCP

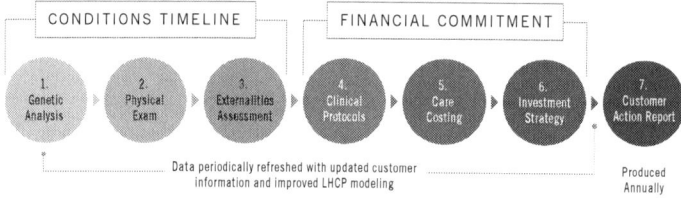

CONDITIONS TIMELINE   FINANCIAL COMMITMENT

1. Genetic Analysis   2. Physical Exam   3. Externalities Assessment   4. Clinical Protocols   5. Care Costing   6. Investment Strategy   7. Customer Action Report

Data periodically refreshed with updated customer information and improved LHCP modeling   Produced Annually

CONDITIONS TIMELINE

The Conditions Timeline is a projection of all the health ailments that an individual is likely to develop over the course of his or her lifetime. Both quantitative and qualitative information feed into the development of this data set. Demographic, epidemiological, and social trends are also incorporated to capture the influence of externalities on a customer's health profile.

1. GENETIC ANALYSIS

The initial component of the LHCP is a genetic assessment. Such an analysis will identify the "hard-coded" health conditions and susceptibilities of the customer. This genetic coding could start at birth, assuming that a guardian will oversee the management and make contributions to the LHCP while the customer is a minor. More likely, at least in the early years of the Dream Plan rollout, the LHCP would be initiated upon adulthood.

Biotechnology research in genetics has exploded over the past decade. Companies like 23andMe and Ancestry.com offer consumer-based services to learn about an individual's genetic composition. It has become common for physicians to recommend genetic testing to determine our susceptibility for certain types of cancers or other conditions as a regular part of our annual well checks.

Already, access to this information influences patient behavior with regard to preventive and proactive treatments. For example, some women who test positive for a mutation in the BRCA 1 or BRCA 2 genes, which indicates an aggressive and often deadly form of breast cancer, opt for a double mastectomy. Imagine how Americans might behave if they knew everything about their genetic profiles.

As part of the Genetic Analysis, individuals would provide blood samples and, depending on the sophistication of the testing capabilities, other biological matter, to enable detailed testing to be conducted. As the years progress, the breadth and depth of genetic testing will expand. Over time, the LHCP should incorporate these advancements and update its projections to provide customers with more refined information.

The genetic testing module would also ask for data about family members. Such information is usually provided from memory and may not be completely comprehensive or accurate. Individuals who have been adopted may not have access to this information. Nonetheless, certain factors, such as the age and cause of death of parents, can be very useful in improving an assessment of a customer's genetic profile.

2. PHYSICAL EXAM

A strong physician/patient relationship is an essential component to the Dream Plan (for both LHCP holders and for public health enrollees). Data from an annual physical such as height, weight, blood pressure, and heart rate would be collected. This would be enhanced with information about cholesterol readings, hormone levels, and whatever else might be clinically relevant to the customer's health.

A Physical Exam should be completed every year. Identifying historical trends in data is an important input into projections about a customer's future health. Individuals who suddenly gain weight or whose bloodwork comes back from the lab with abnormal readings could be demonstrating early indicators for health conditions that the LHCP estimates they may develop. Proactively managing these symptoms before they advance will significantly enhance a customer's health status.

In addition, the annual incorporation of health information ensures that the LHCP serves as a dynamic, regularly updated tool. The data provided by the LHCP should change and evolve as the customer's health status (and as noted next, behaviors) evolves. Providing the customer with continuously updated information should keep them engaged in positive behaviors that maintain or improve their health for the decades they'll be participating in an LHCP.

3. EXTERNALITIES ASSESSMENT

This assessment captures the nonclinical factors that influence an individual's health. It would have a component that includes demographic data such as marital status, address, occupation, salary, and education level. Sociologists, epidemiologists, and other scientists who develop the LHCP will be able to use these factors to project health outcomes.

Customer behaviors will also need to be captured. Data about a customer's diet and exercise regimens are essential, as these behaviors feature strongly in the longitudinal outcomes of an individual. Some LHCPs may collect the information through a customer survey, which may simply ask them to complete a periodic questionnaire. Other LHCPs may be a little more invasive and scour an individual's social media accounts to collect information. Customers may agree to wear devices like Fitbits or other IOT (Internet of Things) wearable contraptions that capture biometric information. Depending on the device and the apps, other helpful data, like information about sleeping habits or stress levels, could also be collected.

More challenging will be the ability to truthfully capture the so-called "sinful habits" related to activities like smoking, drinking, drugs, gambling, and risky sexual behavior. The more culturally unacceptable the behavior is, the less likely the individual is to share it. Yet many of these factors can significantly impact health outcomes. Customers should be aware that the more forthcoming they are in sharing this information, the more precise the projections in the LHCP will be.

Alternatively, LHCP companies should recognize that many LHCP customers will never share certain types of behavior because the risks in doing so outweigh the benefits. An airline pilot who shares his recreational enjoyment of cocaine could lose his job should the information inadvertently be shared with his employer. A woman with multiple sexual partners could ruin her marriage if she feels her data will not be held securely in the LHCP.

Herein lies one opportunity for LHCP companies to differentiate themselves. Some companies may be able to develop personality behavioral profiles based on some of the inputs collected in their LHCP accounts. Such profiles would require considerable research on the myriad factors that contribute to risky behavior and would require leading-edge professional and technological sophistication in their development. The cost to create such profiles may be significant. But if the results justify the means, meaning if the accuracy of the LHCP is significantly improved due to the incorporation of such tools, then the market will determine an acceptable price for the solution.

OUTPUT OF THE CONDITIONS TIMELINE

Data from the Genetic Analysis, the Physical Exam, and the Externalities Assessment are the building blocks to determine the Conditions Timeline. This report will identify the diseases and conditions that an individual will develop during their lifetime.

Generating the Conditions Timeline is the most challenging component of the LHCP because it is an entirely predictive model that will vary from person to person. The accuracy with which different companies will determine their customers' Conditions Timelines will be a key point of product differentiation.

At the beginning of the LHCP process, new customers will meet with LHCP professionals to discuss the outputs of the Conditions Timeline and of the Financial Commitment. Both of these reports will have baseline information that should be discussed in detail. In particular, LHCP companies should develop protocols to ensure that sensitive and potentially life-altering information that is determined through the Conditions Timeline analysis is communicated to the customers with compassion and privacy.

Imagine the shock that you might feel if you, a celebrated college athlete, were going to develop multiple sclerosis in your forties and wind up wheelchair-bound by your fiftieth birthday. In a different scenario, you may learn that the bloodwork collected as part of your Physical Exam revealed that you have a genetic mutation that skips generations. You don't have it, but you've probably passed it along to your kids. A balance of medical professionals, counselors, and LHCP personnel should be either present or available to customers when sensitive LHCP information is being discussed.

Undoubtedly, some serious ethical questions will have to be addressed as more and more individuals enroll in LHCPs. For example, some individuals may not want to know the details of their Conditions Timeline. They may just want the recommendations about what behavioral modifications they should undertake to ensure that they are doing the best that they possibly can to maintain their health. If the individual is capable of saving enough money to pay for the conditions identified in the Timeline, then he or she may be even less interested in learning the specifics of his or her future health status.

LHCP companies would have to be legally protected from any action that could result from *not* communicating life-threatening information about a customer to that customer. Let's say you are a risk-taker and decide to take out loans to buy a home or start a business. Now consider what would happen if you developed an aggressive form of cancer and died the following year. Your beneficiaries could assume considerable debt due to this sad and sudden outcome.

Now let's consider that your Conditions Timeline had predicted that cancer, but you had declined the option to learn about it. The LHCP company cannot be held responsible for the actions you took or for the decisions you made. This is but one of many situations that will arise as LHCPs are adapted and Conditions Timelines are developed for their customers.

FINANCIAL COMMITMENT

The Financial Commitment takes all the inputs from the Conditions Timeline to create a financial plan for the customer. The output of the Financial Commitment is an approach to investing that will match the needs and capabilities of the customer. As will be discussed, the initial Financial Commitment report may require the customer to modify some of his or her preferences about the expected levels of savings they'll need to set aside or about the amount of health care services he or she plans to utilize.

4. CLINICAL PROTOCOLS

The Conditions Timetable identifies what illnesses a customer will get and when. Clinical Protocols specify the treatments that will be required to care for the customer. Treatments and medications for illnesses will be identified. Preventive care activities to promote wellness will also be outlined.

Let's assume your Conditions Timeline determined that you have a high probability of developing prostate cancer. Preventive screenings will be incorporated at intervals that have the best chance of identifying the cancer before it spreads. This is a key advantage to having a Conditions Timeline. Instead of relying on timetables for screenings that average Americans use, your timetable will be customized to your health needs.

A conservative LHCP model would assume that the screenings would be unable to catch the cancer before treatment was necessary. Therefore, a protocol of doctor visits, tests, procedures, and treatments would be included in the Clinical Protocols plan to address the issue. Other requirements, such as recommended pharmaceuticals and even mental health support, would be outlined too.

Clinical Protocols will vary from patient to patient, disease to disease, and doctor to doctor. The LHCP should include standard protocols recommended by industry clinicians and organizations like the AMA, CMS, and any specialty-specific groups like the American Academy of Orthopaedic Surgeons for orthopedics or the

American College of Obstetricians and Gynecologists for women's health. This baseline is a good starting point for customers to use in discussions with their primary care doctor as well as any other relevant clinicians when they are considering a care plan that best suits their needs.

Baseline protocols can be supplemented with alternative information. Benchmark data from other LHCP users of a similar background to a particular customer could be used as a point of comparison. The standard clinical baseline may result in a customer over or under budgeting for care when they compare themselves to like individuals. As the LHCP market grows, this comparison data will become extraordinarily valuable in helping to determine the optimal treatment plans for different types of individuals.

Additionally, alternative treatment options could be presented. An individual suffering from back pain may be recommended to undergo surgery based on the baseline clinical protocol. The patient may be averse to opting for a surgical procedure as a first option and might want to consider less invasive alternatives. The individual might opt to enroll in a weight loss program or utilize massage to address their concerns with back pain.

Customizing the care plan may require medical professionals to counsel patients on the impact and efficacy of their choices because some individuals may select care preferences that significantly diverge from standard industry practices. An example may be a customer who's expected to develop cancer. This individual may decline the recommended chemotherapy in favor of acupuncture. The customer must be made aware of the risks of planning for a less proven treatment plan. Some medical professionals may not even sign off on such protocols. The relative power over establishing care protocols will be a give-and-take between physicians and customers. This is another ethical quandary that will flare up as LHCPs are adopted.

Family members must also be part of the conversation. As with all aspects of the LHCP, the Clinical Protocols will evolve as a customer gets older. As the years progress, customers should be thinking critically about their end-of-life plans. Legal documents, such as power of attorney and do not resuscitate (DNR) orders, should be in place to make sure that the plan that was developed can be implemented with the support of family and friends as the individual ages.

5. CARE COSTING

An important component of the Dream Plan is that customers will pay providers directly for health care services. There will no longer be an insurance intermediary in the form of a commercial company or the government (at least as far as LHCP customers are concerned). Providers will have to establish prices for their health care services, and these prices will need to be made publicly available so consumers can shop and compare.

This will be a radical change from how health care services are procured today. As discussed, Medicare sets the rates it pays providers for care. Commercial insurance companies usually pay providers a different rate, which is often higher than the government's rate. Medicaid is considered the industry's lowest payer. Reimbursement for these cases and even many Medicare cases often does not cover provider costs. The doctor or hospital must rely on the payments from patients with higher-paying private insurance to make up the difference. In other words, at least from a variable cost basis, payments from private insurers ostensibly subsidize the care delivered to patients enrolled in most government-funded health care programs.

That doesn't mean that providers can't drive down their costs. There's always room for improvement. Value-based care efforts and other pay-for-performance models have had some success in reducing costs in today's system. But the model has its limitations. Direct-to-provider payments offer a lot of potential to "right size" the prices of health care goods and services.

The direct-pay model has gained some ground in health care, but market-based prices are far from the industry norm. There's little incentive for most providers to create market-based prices because they're typically paid by insurers, not individuals. And as noted in our discussion about the emergency room, hospitals are creating bills off of charge master rates, not market-tested prices, when they charge many patients for care.

Yet some market-based pricing is available in health care. Cash-to-provider payments are made in primary care, at stand-alone urgent care clinics or regional chains like MedSpring. Retailers such as Walmart, as well as pharmacy outlets like CVS and Walgreens, are all starting to offer some sort of cash-based primary care service. There are retail lab companies, like Any Lab Test Now, that can conduct many lab tests on site too.

Some ambulatory surgery centers (ASCs) also offer services on a retail basis. This is becoming more common as more Americans enroll in high-deductible health plans (HDHP). As with any insurance plan, an individual with a HDHP must pay the entire deductible before the insurer will pay for their portion of the care. At issue is the fact that the cost of some surgeries and procedures, like colonoscopies, is often-times lower than the amount of the deductible. Since that patient will have to pay out of pocket for the procedure, they are incented to shop around and find the best deal they can. That's one reason why more ASCs are offering such direct-pay terms of service.

ASCs are a great site for retail pricing because the majority of the costs of service are easily identifiable. By definition, cases done in the outpatient environment are lower risk, and they are less complicated than what's done in a hospital. That means there is less variability in the care that's delivered, making it fairly straightforward to iden-tify a reasonable price. In fact, some ASCs only take cash. A pioneer in this area is the Surgery Center of Oklahoma in Oklahoma City. They've been providing market-based, direct-to-consumer pricing for years.[1]

In the short term, a key source of pricing for services will be claims databases. The information in these databases is a consolidation of rates that different providers are paid for different services by differ-ent payers. It's like a clearinghouse of all the charges and payments in different communities around the country. The data is available to the public through websites like healthcarebluebook.com. More detailed information can be purchased from organizations like Truven Health Analytics. LHCP companies will probably utilize data from claims databases in conjunction with rates from local providers to determine Care Costing in the LHCP.

As for pharmaceuticals, pricing today is extraordinarily complicated, as most drug manufacturers do not sell their products to the general public on a retail basis. But maybe they should, and perhaps they will. A number of strategies outlined in the next chapter may help LHCP members gain access to drugs at reasonable rates. LHCP designers and industry advocates will need to continue to pressure Big Pharma to be more transparent with pricing. In the meantime, data about selected drugs that can be used to populate the LHCP is available through sites such as goodrx.com and online claims databases.

6. INVESTMENT STRATEGY

The LHCP investment team will use the inputs from the prior modules to develop an investment plan for the customer. The sophistication with which these plans are designed can be yet another differentiator between LHCP companies. The more returns a company can generate from an LHCP customer's investments, the less money the individual will need to save to fund their care.

As with any long-term investment, LHCP customers may be encouraged to invest as much money as possible as early as possible. Early contributions can grow the LHCP asset base more quickly which allows for higher returns on investments over a long period of time. This security can help overcome the many financial challenges in life, from a loss of a job to a divorce. Customers will also be advised that any money left in the LHCP can be willed to beneficiaries. Such knowledge may incent customers to be more conservative with their investments.

From the costing side, new therapies or drugs might be developed that can prevent the onset of or cure diseases that a customer may develop. When these advancements are introduced to the market, customers should discuss these options with medical professionals to determine if they should be incorporated into their care plan. Such decisions will update the Conditions Timeline because the disease a customer was expected to develop will now have a cure. In turn, the Investment Strategy should also update, ensuring that the customer's financial commitments will cover the cost of these new therapies, drugs, or procedures.

OUTPUT OF THE FINANCIAL COMMITMENT

As discussed, LHCP companies will need to have consultative sessions with customers once their Conditions Timelines and Financial Commitments are complete. When consulting with customers about their Financial Commitments, advisers will explain how much money the individual will need to contribute. Financial planners may present customers with multiple options depending on their current financial position. Individuals with high incomes may be encouraged to invest more money earlier, either through a significant lump-sum payment or through higher periodic payments in the short term than required in the long term. Those with tight financial resources may be given very specific guidelines regarding their expected contributions and may be provided with only one option for investing.

In some cases, the conversations may require the input of medical professionals too, particularly if the clinical pathway designed by the customer is too expensive for them to afford. The medical professional can help identify "niceties" that the customer may have added but are not critical to their long-term well-being. For example, a customer may have budgeted for weekly acupuncture sessions to address the stress associated with their job. Changing the frequency of the sessions to monthly rather than weekly may allow for the reallocation of a high enough level of payments to address the shortfall in the customer's financial need.

If the gap is too significant to be addressed with minor modifications to the care plan, the customer will still have options. As will be discussed, individuals may try to increase their income or reduce their financial requirement by taking steps to improve their long-term health. Ultimately, any individual who does not have the resources to pay for the care they need will default into the public health pool. Details on public health in the Dream Plan are covered in chapter 12.

CUSTOMER ACTION REPORT

Once the customer has reviewed the baseline data in the Conditions Timeline and has committed to the funding requirements outlined in the Financial Commitment, the LHCP provider can create a baseline Customer Action Report (CAR). The CAR will become the annual report that customers review with their LHCP representatives. Each year, customers will complete their physicals and update their behavioral analyses. The LHCP company will update the LHCP and identify any changes to the Conditions Timeline and to the Financial Commitment required of the customer. Individuals will learn if their health has improved or gotten worse, if they are on target with their savings, and how these changes impact their future health and financial position.

So many of the health problems that plague Americans—from obesity to hypertension to different types of cancers—can be prevented. A key component of a CAR will be the identification of preventive action that the customer can engage in to forestall or prevent the onset of projected diseases and conditions. Doing so can take a potential funding gap problem that many LHCP applicants will face and turn it into a health improvement opportunity. These individuals may try to make behavioral modifications to improve their health, thereby reducing their financial obligations to sustainable levels.

Common recommendations will be weight loss, stress reduction, and increased exercise. More patient-specific recommendations are likely to be identified as the individual grows older and more data about the individual's behavioral history and health outcomes are identified. Importantly, the CAR gives the LHCP customer the ability to meaningfully improve their future health by modifying their behavior today. The opportunity to live a healthier, more productive life should be all the incentive that anyone needs to commit to enhanced wellness activities.

LHCP PROFITABILITY MODEL

The LHCP differs from other proposals to transform the health care industry in one critical way: It enables the managers of the LHCP products to make money. Customers may access LHCPs in the same way as when they would open an investment account with a financial services entity. They'll give the investing company their money to be saved over a long period of time. In exchange for holding the cash and generating a positive return, the investing company takes a fee. Collecting these and other potential fees would be the revenue stream that would enable the LHCP companies to be profitable.

Of course, an LHCP provider would be doing much more than simply investing money. They will be performing genetic testing, conducting proprietary research and data analysis, ensuring data security, coordinating with doctors and enrollees, and interacting with the health care system in a completely new way. Initially, the costs to create and manage such an enterprise will be high. But costs should come down as adaption of the products increases.

Just how these LHCP companies decide to charge the enrollees could vary significantly. A flat, up-front fee could be charged to the customer to pay for the initial testing and background assessments. The company could charge an additional fee to be collected periodically, which may depend on the amount of dollars invested in an individual's LHCP.

LHCP managers could generate tangential revenue streams by vertically integrating into the health care delivery environment. For example, the recommendations in a CAR could result in a referral to a weight loss clinic. The LHCP company could get a fee for the referral. In fact, the LHCP company could be a full or part owner in the company that administers the weight loss program. Of course, any conflict of interest in making such a referral would have to be avoided in order to ensure that the LHCP company remains unbiased in its recommendations.

Customers saving money for health care costs may also be saving money for retirement. LHCP companies could generate incremental fees if they wind up doing both LHCP and retirement planning for these individuals. LHCP providers may offer the customer a discount on the rate for retirement planning, given that they will already have an established relationship with the customer for the LHCP business.

CHAPTER 9

THE OBSOLESCENCE
OF TRADITIONAL
HEALTH INSURANCE

Ever wonder why you can't buy health insurance from the same company that insures your car or your home? The reason is simple. Health insurance isn't just insurance. It provides a variety of benefits that have little to do with giving us coverage against the unexpected, unpredictable events in life that pure insurance programs are all about.

Today, health plans must comply with complicated regulatory burdens. As discussed, ACA plans must offer ten essential benefits, a comprehensive package of services that includes coverage for what are considered basic needs. Employer-sponsored health plans also offer robust coverage. Employers do this as a means to attract employees, and can offer not only all the options included in the ACA's ten essential benefits requirement, but also coverage for services like chiropractic visits, massage, and acupuncture. As a result, health insurance is not a risk-based product like car insurance. It's more of a hybrid catch-as-catch-can of benefits, all tucked under a broad payment plan that creates price opacity and inefficiency.

The LHCP provides customers with an incredible wealth of information about their future health conditions. Such data invalidates the need for a product that insures against every conceivable health care interaction that an individual might have with the system. The Dream Plan renders traditional health insurance obsolete. The LHCP eliminates many of the unknown events that may affect its customers and, better yet, articulates the kinds of things they'll need to plan for.

Today's health insurance models focus on covering clinical benefits, like hospital care and ER services. The Dream Plan takes a different tact. It breaks down the customer's coverage requirements into functional benefits. Functional benefits refer to how the insurance or coverage is supposed to work, not the specific clinical service that the patient might utilize. This shift is important because it allows for LHCP designers to develop payment models and funding mechanisms that match each type of functional benefit. Customer dollars can be much more efficiently used, which will lower the cost of health care in America.

Right now, health insurance offers what could be regarded as five different functional benefits: primary, periodic, chronic, catastrophic, and incapacitation. These benefits vary by functional category based on the frequency that Americans access them and the cost per episode of care.

CHART 11. SPECTRUM OF FUNCTIONAL BENEFITS

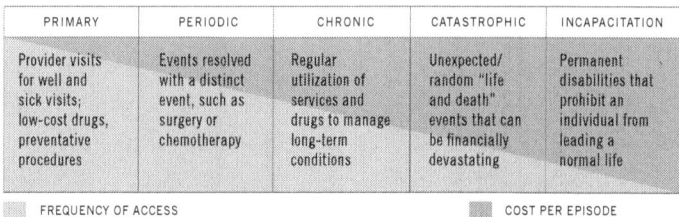

PRIMARY	PERIODIC	CHRONIC	CATASTROPHIC	INCAPACITATION
Provider visits for well and sick visits; low-cost drugs, preventative procedures	Events resolved with a distinct event, such as surgery or chemotherapy	Regular utilization of services and drugs to manage long-term conditions	Unexpected/ random "life and death" events that can be financially devastating	Permanent disabilities that prohibit an individual from leading a normal life

FREQUENCY OF ACCESS   COST PER EPISODE

As with many strategic models, high-volume activities typically require a lower per-unit cost, and low-volume functions accessed by fewer people have a higher cost. This dynamic applies to the Spectrum of Functional Benefits, too.

Primary care is a functional benefit characterized by a high frequency of visits, and each of these visits has a relatively low per-unit cost. These are high-volume services for a number of reasons. Primary care is used to address the most basic health needs that impact every American. Visits to a PCP or lab for blood tests, treatment for minor health concerns, and education about preventive health services are all primary care services. In addition, primary care acts as the gateway to other, more complex services, which drives up the frequency of these encounters.

At the other end of the spectrum lie catastrophic care and permanent incapacitation. These categories are very high cost and affect a small percentage of Americans. These are cases where an individual has sustained a significant health issue that impedes his or her ability to function normally or independently. Severe strokes, paralysis, and degenerative diseases fall into these categories. Not surprisingly, the cost to treat these cases is significant.

Periodic care and chronic care lie in the middle of the Spectrum of Functional Benefits. Periodic care includes discrete episodes and therapies, such as surgeries or prescriptive rehabilitation. We will all have periodic episodes of care throughout our lives. These encounters may be somewhat expensive on a per-unit basis, but they have distinct start and end points. That makes the financial risk associated with them lower than some other forms of care because the costs for treatment can be well defined.

Chronic care relates to the drugs and therapies that are required to manage lifelong conditions. The costs associated with managing chronic care can be somewhat low on a per-unit basis, but their duration of need makes the overall cost to manage a chronic condition high. Not all Americans have a chronic condition, meaning that fewer Americans will access these services compared with those for primary or periodic care.

Using the LHCP to break out health insurance into functional benefits allows for the creation of a system that matches a distinct funding model to each of the five benefits. LHCP designers can right size how customer dollars are invested based on the functional benefits they'll need. For example, the low-cost/high-volume interactions that characterize primary care would be paid in cash, eliminating many of the administrative costs associated with the contracting, billing, and paying of these events. Individuals would use traditional risk-based insurance (like car insurance that insures against an accident) for catastrophic issues since they'd be insuring against the unknown, unpredictable events that an LHCP can't plan for. As will be described, other funding mechanisms could be used for the different functional benefits, depending on the customer.

PRIMARY CARE: TODAY AND IN THE DREAM PLAN

TODAY

Much of primary care is consultative. It does not require expensive equipment or complicated therapies. Many primary care interactions can and are being done virtually through telemedicine and other technologically enabled means of communication. As a result, the cost for a primary care interaction is relatively inexpensive.

Primary care is critically important, misunderstood, and underutilized in today's health care model. Primary care physicians should be trusted, long-term partners in ensuring the health and well-being of patients. This enables the physician to develop protocols and clinical recommendations that best match a patient's needs and lifestyle.

Unfortunately, many patients do not have such a stable, trusted relationship with their primary care provider. In fact, many people don't even know who their primary care doctor is. If a patient gets sick, they're more than likely to take the first available appointment in the PCP's office—and that may not be with their doctor. They may see a nurse, who is qualified to test and diagnose common conditions like the flu and bronchitis. Some health plans allow patients to see specialists without a PCP referral. This further limits contact between the patient and the PCP.

The current health insurance system has transformed the primary care physician's role from a problem-solving partner to an administrative gatekeeper and a fever, bumps, and bruises diagnostician. It's one of the reasons that fewer and fewer medical school students are focusing on primary care. The work isn't as stimulating as it used to be, and the pay is much lower than it is for other specialties.[1] By 2025, estimates indicate that there will be a shortage of about 35,000 primary care doctors around the country. Such a shortage will impede not only access to care, but also the quality of care in America.

DREAM PLAN

In the Dream Plan, patients will have the opportunity to select a provider of their choosing—not just the ones preapproved by an insurer or by the government. Customers will pay primary care providers directly for the care they receive. Paying for the service is one way to ensure that a customer can derive value from the experience. Direct payment should increase patient engagement, which in turn has been shown to improve outcomes.[2]

The cost for many primary care services, although comparatively low, would be built into the LHCP. Primary care includes not only an office visit, but also lab work and other diagnostic tests. Many consider preventive care, such as preventive mammograms and colonoscopies, under the primary care umbrella, too. Should a patient's LHCP indicate that such diagnostic tests be required, they would be included in the Clinical Protocols at recommended intervals. The cost for these tests would be budgeted into the Financial Commitment so customers will have the cash on hand to pay for these encounters when they need to. Yet some of the primary care encounters, such as those for sniffles and fevers, should be paid in cash out of pocket.

In fact, an annual primary care visit is so important that it is considered mandatory in the Dream Plan. All Americans, whether they have an LHCP or are on public health, would be required to have one. The annual visit for LHCP holders ensures that their vitals (height, weight, blood pressure) and other key metrics from bloodwork and diagnostic tests are entered into their Conditions Timelines. Doing so maintains the robustness of the individual's data set, which, in turn, can improve the predictive capabilities of the LHCP.

PERIODIC CARE: TODAY AND IN THE DREAM PLAN

TODAY

Periodic care refers to the different health care issues that occur regularly throughout one's life and are relatively inexpensive to fund. This category includes events or clusters of events that have a discrete start and end period. These issues are what may be termed "closed" in that they are diagnosed, treated, and resolved as best as can be expected. Treatment ends, and the patient does not return to see the doctor because the health condition has been addressed.

For example, a periodic condition relates to the activities required to address a torn ligament. The individual may need surgery or simply a cast. Rehabilitation may be necessary. All of these costs would be part of the periodic event. Once the ligament is healed, the patient reaches clinical resolution. In some cases, the individual may not heal completely, but no other treatments can improve their condition. While the patient may not return to their former lifestyle, the periodic event is considered closed.

Periodic care can also be the result of the culmination of a chronic condition. Cancer is sometimes considered a chronic condition. Patients who require chemotherapy to treat malignant growths only require the therapy for a determined period of time. Therefore, chemotherapy would be considered a periodic treatment. Any subsequent lifelong drugs that the patient might need would fall under chronic care and will be discussed in the next section.

The cost of periodic care can run from about one thousand to tens of thousands of dollars, depending on the issue. For example, a more complicated periodic episode, such as a total knee replacement, might run anywhere between under $20,000 to over $70,000.[3] (The Surgery Center of Oklahoma, which offers strictly cash-based pricing, lists the base price for a knee replacement at a little over $15,000.) Pricing at the high end of the spectrum is reflective of today's prices, which should come down considerably in the Dream Plan. The ultimate price would depend on the health status of the patient (whether they are young or old, overweight, have other health conditions), the implant used for the knee replacement, the location of the surgery, the surgeon performing the care, etc. Other periodic concerns, such as the removal of a malignant skin lesion, should cost well under $2,500.[4]

DREAM PLAN

The LHCP will provide all the funding that's necessary to cover periodic health conditions that may occur in an individual's life. Because these episodes of care are closed, financial planners can be fairly confident in understanding the dollar amounts that should be reserved to pay for these conditions. That said, some periodic events will be easier to cost out than others. Cataract surgery is much less complicated than a craniotomy. Cost estimators will have some idea of the expenses associated with brain surgery, but the potential for variability is high given the complex nature of the procedure. LHCP financial planners will have to account for a range of costs for some periodic events.

One of the challenges with funding periodic care relates to timing of unexpected events. These are different than catastrophic events (which are described later). The odds that the periodic event will happen are very high, so the LHCP will budget for the care required to address it. But it's unexpected because the timing of when the event may occur is difficult to pinpoint. If the event occurs sooner than expected in the Conditions Timeline, the requisite money may not be available to pay for the care at the time of the incident.

An example is an individual who is an avid mountain biker. This is a sport where participants have a high likelihood of sustaining personal injury. Based on an individual's age, fitness level, experience with the sport, and frequency of participation, the LHCP will account for some type of expected injury.

Let's say our mountain biker breaks his collarbone at age thirty-one. The individual might need consultations with an orthopedist, imaging, pain medication, rehabilitation, and/or a host of other clinical treatments. This care should not be in excess of $10,000 and, in fact, should be much lower (assuming no surgery is required).

The design of each LHCP will ensure that cash is available for selected preventive health care needs at each stage of a person's life. But the program will also require that a certain amount of capital is kept in reserve strictly for investment purposes. The more money that is invested early in an individual's life, the more potential it has to grow over a longer period of time.

By thirty-one, our mountain biker should have saved more than $10,000 in an LHCP. Yet taking $10,000 out of the LHCP investment fund at this point in his life causes the individual to forego the significant investment upside that the money could generate later. In thirty years, with a 6% growth rate, $10,000 could become about $60,000.

It may make more financial sense for the mountain biker to take out a loan to address the collarbone problem. The money in the LHCP would serve as collateral for a lender (which could also be the organization that operates the LHCP). The mountain biker can then consult with the investment team managing the LHCP to determine the optimal means by which to pay off the loan while continuing to invest in his future health care needs.

CHRONIC CARE: TODAY AND IN THE DREAM PLAN

TODAY

Chronic conditions are persistent, long-lasting conditions and diseases. A chronic condition may be considered as such if it lasts longer than three months. Examples include Alzheimer's and dementia, arthritis, asthma, depression, diabetes, HIV-AIDS, and high blood pressure. Chronic conditions range in how they may impact one's daily life. Symptoms of some conditions seemingly never abate, causing the patient continuous pain or discomfort. Other symptoms flare up and go into remission. How different individuals develop chronic disease will depend on a variety of factors. Some conditions are causes for others (like high cholesterol can cause diabetes). Some can be contracted (like HIV-AIDS), while others result from one's genetic makeup (autism, schizophrenia).

Chronic conditions typically require long-term or lifetime costs to manage the treatment of the symptoms or the condition itself. Diabetics require insulin. Those suffering from depression may require medication and/or therapy. Individuals with chronic obstructive pulmonary disorder (COPD) may need a nebulizer or a source of oxygen to assist in breathing.

The cost to manage some chronic diseases may be relatively low on a per-unit basis. Medication for an HIV patient can run anywhere from less than twenty to over a thousand dollars a pill if a generic option isn't available.[5] The concern, of course, is that the medication is required for the patient's entire life. Estimates put the lifetime cost to treat HIV at over $400,000.[6] This type of expense might force an individual out of an LHCP and into a public health pool simply because the expense, coupled with other expected health care costs, would be too onerous to bear.

DREAM PLAN

Individuals with a diagnosis of a chronic condition may find significant benefit from components of the Dream Plan. Importantly, the Conditions Timeline encourages a physician and a patient to manage the holistic health of the patient. Such a collaborative approach can provide patients with behavioral modifications that can mitigate, forestall, or even eliminate the development of some chronic conditions. Doing so can improve an individual's health and reduce their financial burden.

Improved diet, weight loss, stress reduction, and exercise are activities that can help address the symptoms of many chronic conditions. Type 2 diabetes is one example. Studies have shown that for certain patients, weight loss has been a contributing factor to eliminating the disease.[7] Improving social interactions and exercise can improve cognitive abilities and delay the onset of dementia and Alzheimer's.[8] One study showed that "grounding"—having physical contact with the earth by engaging in activities such as walking barefoot outside—could help address symptoms of some autoimmune diseases![9]

While behavioral modifications can cure a few chronic diseases and can lessen the impact of symptoms, other therapies may be required. LHCP participants will still have to budget for these costs.

One estimate indicates that 86% of all health care costs are associated with individuals who have one or more chronic condition.[10] Estimates like this include costs captured in different categories of the Spectrum of Functional Benefits, not just those included in chronic care. It's important to change the way we look at what are considered chronic conditions because our current categorization casts a wide net over too many services offered by too many providers in too many locations. It's hard to use the optimal financial mechanism to pay for each of the chronic care costs if they're all lumped together.

The intent in breaking out the costs this way is not to change how physicians treat their patients. Doctors have their work cut out for them treating chronically ill patients, and they can execute their professional charge however they see fit. My intent is to use the money to pay for the care as efficiently as possible. Instead of running all the dollars to pay for the different functional categories of chronic care through the same payment system (which right now is a centralized insurance system run by either the government or private insurers), the Dream Plan separates the costs and funds them in ways better aligned to their magnitude and frequency.

Consider a man with hypertension. A cardiac procedure such as an angioplasty or surgery that is required to address the hypertension would *not* be considered a chronic care cost in the Dream Plan. The procedure itself is a *periodic* treatment. The drugs and lifelong specialty doctor visits associated with treating hypertension *would* be considered chronic costs. If the hypertension is treated by a patient's primary care doctor, then the provider visits would fall under the primary care category.

That angioplasty required by our customer with hypertension? As described in the previous section, a periodic condition would be paid either through money that accumulated in an LHCP or through a loan. The primary care visits would be paid in cash. The funding for the chronic drug costs could be improved using some new ideas, too.

PHARMACY BENEFITS MANAGER

Today, consumers buy drugs from pharmacies. Pharmacies serve as distribution points for drugs. Distribution companies or pharmacies act as pharmacy benefit managers, or PBMs, by buying the drugs from pharmaceutical companies in bulk. Drug prices are inflated today because there's little to no transparency between the price that the drug company sells the drugs for, and the price the consumer pays for it.

The Dream Plan could cut down on drug prices by creating its own PBM that would negotiate directly with pharmaceutical companies. This separate entity could pay pharmacies to distribute the drugs and establish cash prices that the LHCP members would pay for their medications. Such a cash-to-pharmacy situation would benefit the pharmacy because it could avoid the administrative costs associated with how third-party payment processing is done today. Managing rebates and coupons and tiered pricing for drugs would be simplified in the Dream Plan. Pharmacies would just get cash directly from LHCP members.

Bulk discount negotiations, like those used by a PBM in today's model, require the negotiator to have an idea of how many and what type of drugs their members will need. Predictive analytics in the LHCP can do an excellent job of identifying these volumes because it calculates, by person, who'll need what and when. With the robust data collected in the LHCPs, a third-party organization negotiating drug prices on behalf of the LHCP member community is less likely to overpay by buying too many drugs that don't get used, and it won't get penalized for needing more drugs than it bargained for. Better articulation of the demand for drugs should help bring costs down.

DRUG "ANNUITY" PROGRAM

Creating an LHCP-sponsored PBM could be an effective, although conventional, way to bring down costs in the Dream Plan. Another approach seeks to match the periodic payments for drugs that the chronically ill must expend with a financial instrument that can generate the needed payment. Here's how it would work.

A variety of financial investment products are available that enable individuals to receive payments, or distributions, from an investment they've made. An annuity is a common retirement vehicle that allows the individual to receive periodic payments from a base amount of capital that they've invested. The payment is derived from earnings that the investment accumulated over the years, and it can also be comprised of part of the principal that generates the returns.

In the Dream Plan, drug "annuities" could be created by LHCP companies as a means to fund their customers' chronic drug costs. The financial investment team would design a plan that would ensure that the customer saved enough money for all their health care needs, just like any other LHCP. Yet this plan would be structured in a way that would also enable periodic withdrawals from the plan. Such a financial model would require more capital early in the plan's investment cycle in order to build up the funding necessary to sustain the periodic payments.

It may be challenging for many individuals to fund such a model. They might be able to generate some periodic disbursements, but it might not be enough to cover their chronic drug costs. However, this drug annuity model can and should be used by donors and charity organizations as a means to help supplement drug costs for the sick.

Consider the creation of a drug annuity for HIV-AIDS patients. Right now, myriad fund-raising efforts are in operation that collect money to help find a cure for the virus, increase education about treatment and prevention, and subsidize the costs and/or pay for the treatment for certain individuals. It is in this latter area where a drug annuity program could have a more powerful impact.

Rather than being used to provide direct subsidies for individuals, donations would be channeled to the central annuity fund. The fund could even be endowed by wealthy sponsors with a personal connection to the disease. Think of what would happen if the Elton John AIDS Foundation used some of its capital for the sole purpose of subsidizing the drug costs for HIV-AIDS sufferers in an LHCP fund. As the donations to the fund would increase, more and more subsidies could be paid out to qualifying individuals. While this may be how some large foundations structure their resources today, the Dream Plan would demand more transparency on how the dollars are invested and distributed. This is an approach that could be used for LHCP members only and/or could be used in the public health arena to restructure the payment model for chronic drug costs.

CATASTROPHIC CARE: TODAY AND IN THE DREAM PLAN

TODAY

Each of us faces the risk of being impacted by a catastrophic event. We may be in a terrible car accident, struck by lightning, or simply conk our head on the sharp corner of a table at just the right angle to cause a brain injury. These are not the sort of events that can be predicted. These are freak accidents. In some cases, we will go through our entire life and not experience such an event. But if we do, we may be confronted with medical bills that could be financially devastating.

Insurance is tailor-made for catastrophic coverage. Homeowner's insurance is a great example of how catastrophic insurance is used by millions of Americans today. This type of coverage can include clauses for catastrophic events, such as fire and flooding. No doubt the odds of these events occurring are higher in some locations than in others, but homeowners aren't expecting that a seismic event will swallow their three-bedroom ranch and all their belongings with it. But if it does, the homeowner will receive a payment commensurate with the terms and conditions of their homeowner's insurance policy.

Today's health insurance isn't just for catastrophic care. Health insurance covers all kinds of functions. An annual visit to a primary care doctor has nothing to do with providing coverage for an individual who gets struck by lightning. Yet these and many other services are bundled together, obscuring the costs and value of the different services.

Another challenge with budgeting the costs for truly catastrophic insurance with regular health coverage is that health insurance is not completely transferable. Consider an individual who gets mauled by a bear in Montana but has health insurance from their home state of Nevada. Health insurance is required to cover emergency services anywhere in the United States. An ambulance ride and the ER visit in Montana should be covered by the Nevada insurance.

The financial problem comes if the patient requires any nonemergency care. A hospitalization may not be considered emergency care, even if it resulted from an emergency event. The Nevada insurer may cover part of the care, but the patient may not have access to the negotiated, proprietary rates that their insurer could provide for in-network care in Nevada. The patient would have to pay out-of-network rates in Montana. And if those rates are determined by the overinflated charge master, our Nevada friend could be in some serious trouble (aside from the mauling injury). This makes absolutely no sense, because the whole point of catastrophic insurance is that one can predict neither what will happen nor where.

DREAM PLAN

The Dream Plan's predictive capabilities invalidate the need for most traditional insurance. Since the LHCP will make predictions about the future, there isn't all that much to insure. Instead, catastrophic insurance in the Dream Plan focuses on health care costs derived from things that *can't* be predicted.

Today's health insurance focuses on covering the clinical services required—the hospital care, the ER services—if an individual has a catastrophic event. There are so many variables related to how and where care would be delivered in a truly unexpected event. Further, individuals will often need resources to pay for more than just medical care.

Catastrophic insurance under the Dream Plan would be structured on cash distribution levels. Individuals would buy into plans to ensure that they would get a certain payout, say, one hundred thousand dollars' worth of coverage. Assuming the event is catastrophic per the rules of the plan, the funds the customer would receive could be used toward relief of any medical expenses associated with the freak accident. Alternatively, the money might be used to replace property damaged in the accident or to provide interim home care to support the victim. All of these terms and conditions would be hashed out as these products are brought to market.

In the Dream Plan, individuals would be paying direct to provider for services. That means that the cost of care in the Montana hospital that treats the patient who was mauled by the bear will be the same whether the patient lives in Nevada or Montana. The insurance payout would be 100% transferable. Members wouldn't have to worry about where they were if an unforeseen event would happen. They would have the peace of mind that health insurance is supposed to provide, knowing that their medical costs would be covered through this new model.

Should a catastrophic event render an individual permanently incapacitated, they would be eligible for coverage under public health programs described in chapter 12.

PERMANENT INCAPACITATION: TODAY AND IN THE DREAM PLAN

TODAY

Individuals categorized as permanently incapacitated require significant medical and pharmaceutical care through the course of their lives. Individuals may be permanently incapacitated from birth. Issues such as cerebral palsy or congenital heart conditions can result in a permanent, oftentimes uncorrectable lifelong condition. Permanent incapacitation can also result from accidents, surgical errors, or can develop over time due to aging and/or environmental factors.

While advancements in health care and technology have improved treatment options for many of these issues, the ability for these individuals to lead normal lives is remote. Serving as a caregiver for the permanently incapacitated is oftentimes beyond the emotional and physical capabilities of the individual's immediate family, adding to the challenges of living with these conditions.

Today, some individuals with serious medical conditions are covered under their family's insurance plan (although many qualify for additional support through public health programs). Such an approach helps subsidize the cost for the permanently incapacitated by using dollars from the healthier members of a program. The problem is that individuals with significant health issues use a disproportionately high share of resources. Insurance plans with such individuals in the mix can be negatively impacted financially, causing them to identify ways to reduce losses that impact other members.

In other cases, insurers seek to control costs by limiting coverage. They may deny treatment if the protocols are deemed experimental or if medical professionals do not believe additional care will improve the condition of the patient. These issues were at the heart of a recent high-profile case of a terminally ill infant from the United Kingdom, Charlie Gard. The British health system denied treatments for the baby, citing the experimental nature of the drugs that might save him, and his deteriorating health. Both President Trump and Pope Francis weighed in on the side of intervention, dragging out the debate.

Ultimately, Charlie Gard was taken off life support shortly before his first birthday.[11]

Cases like these, while not as sensationalized, regularly occur here at home too. When they do, it's easy to demonize the insurer for prioritizing its own financial health over the health of a member. As more and more sophisticated treatments enter the market, from uterine transplants to genetically customized drugs to DNA modification using CRISPR technology, debates about life, ethics, and money will only intensify.

DREAM PLAN

The cost to care for the very sick would devastate almost any family's financial position. Most individuals who are permanently incapacitated are not candidates for an LHCP because the vast majority of families cannot afford the cost of care required. Funding will not be received through insurers, because traditional health insurance will have been phased out in the Dream Plan. Therefore, most of the funding for individuals with severe health issues will fall under the purview of the government.

The public health program will manage the care for low-income Americans and for those afflicted with serious health conditions. Critically, the budgets for these two populations must be managed separately. Dollars that could be spent on the permanently incapacitated could easily consume the entire public health budget. Care for the poor cannot be sacrificed by inequitably distributing funds toward care for the very ill.

Every American should contribute funds toward their health care costs, even if these contributions do not cover all the required expenses. Therefore, families with minors afflicted with severe illness should make contributions toward funding for their child's care. A fair approach would be to require these families to make a contribution at a level comparable to what families with a healthy child would pay. The cost to care for a minor is not significant and should not be burdensome to most families.

Fortunately, funding options besides tax dollars and family contributions are available for individuals suffering from myriad diseases. In fact, almost $133 billion (about 4% of the $3.3 trillion of health care spend) was contributed by other private sources in 2016. Charitable organizations exist for conditions ranging from breast cancer (the Susan G. Komen Foundation) to multiple sclerosis (the Multiple Sclerosis Foundation) to heart disease (the American Heart Association). Many organizations simply advocate for efforts to reduce disease (like education, or lobbying health groups to focus on treating their constituent diseases), while others subsidize the cost of treatment.

Organizations such as Shriners Hospitals for Children and St. Jude Children's Research Hospital pay for the health care of very sick children regardless of the family's ability to pay. Family foundations have also been created to fund the care of different diseases for certain populations.

Unfortunately, not all the dollars that are contributed to foundations and other not-for-profits are used to fund medical care. Money goes toward operating the organizations, which includes costs for salaries and overhead and advertising and lobbyists and a whole host of categories that take money away from the patients who really need it.

There are ways to track the effectiveness of charities, such as the site charitynavigator.org, which provides comparisons of organizations in multiple industries, not just health care. Under its category for Patient and Family Support, which looks at organizations that support those with serious illnesses, 47 of the 296 charities received zero to two stars in a four-star rating system (four being the best). Fewer than 40% of the organizations had a four-star rating.[12] The Dream Plan would provide more clarity on how resources are being used and better coordination between agencies to maximize the amount of dollars that can be spent on individuals with severe health needs.

One way to reduce the administrative overhead associated with charitable organizations is to shift more of their money-raising initiatives to crowdsourcing platforms such as gofundme.com. Sites like these enable families to raise money for catastrophic medical bills or family support services (and almost anything else related to personal financing). Crowdsourcing can provide much more transparency about how donated money is directed to the needy.

Even better, the funding campaigns can be customized to the individual. Some individuals may be able to use crowdsourcing to provide them with enough funds in an LHCP that will allow them to fund the care they want, given their disability. Allowing these individuals to have more choice in what kind of care they receive and how they will access it can be incredibly empowering—and will probably improve their health. That would be a dream for them and for their families.

CONCLUSION

Given the wealth of options available to treat the variety of diseases and conditions that can afflict any one of us, we should use the resources we have as efficiently as possible. An innovative aspect of the Dream Plan is that it matches the way individuals save their money and pay for care with the functional type of care they'll need: Cash for low-cost, primary care treatment. Insurance for unexpected health calamities. Loans (if necessary) to fund outpatient surgeries and other periodic health events. Annuity-type models that throw off cash to pay for chronic drug costs. Crowdfunding and better coordinated donations for those who are permanently incapacitated. LHCP designers and their customers will incorporate each of these methods as necessary into their longitudinal savings plan to fund their care.

Financial services: Meet health care.

CHAPTER 10

BUSINESS CASE
FOR THE LHCP

The LHCP serves as an investment account to be used by customers to pay for the health care goods and services they'll need over the course of their lives. Customers can fund the account in different ways, although most customers are likely to contribute some of the funds on a periodic, monthly basis. In the Dream Plan, the accountability for funding an individual's lifetime health care expenses falls on the individual, not on the government and not on insurance companies.

Americans don't pay for their health care this way today. Transitioning from today's complicated payment system to the simplified LHCP model will require a seismic shift in the way Americans think about health care spending. The key concern potential customers will have is whether they will be able to save enough money to fund an LHCP or not.

The lack of cost transparency in our current health care system has inhibited most of us from appreciating how much money we actually contribute to the system today, who collects it, and what it's spent on. Each of us should have a lot more comfort with the idea of an LHCP once we better understand these factors.

The "business case" described in this chapter is not an outline of the potential revenue projections and operational costs associated with developing the LHCP product. Rather, it seeks to answer a key strategic question: In today's health care system, does the amount of money contributed by an average American and their employer approximate what is spent per person on health care? If the answer is "yes," then there should be a strong expectation that Americans should be able to use comparable funds in the future to pay for their care in the Dream Plan. In other words, the business case relates to proving, at a very high level, that Americans should be able to finance their own care in a new payment system, especially if that payment system supports a lower-cost, more-efficient health care delivery model.

The business case captures the different ways that a typical American contributes money into the health care system today. It then evaluates the challenges related to redirecting these dollars away from either insurers, the government, or an individual's savings account and into an LHCP. Depending on the reader's background, this analysis is either an overly simplified or incredibly complicated study. A detailed chart with the calculations, data explanations, and sources is included in the LHCP Business Case Detail section at the end of this book.

By no means do the assumptions apply to the vast majority of Americans. Yet any analysis of this nature must begin with some high-level, documented assumptions to prove or disprove the question about health care affordability. This analysis is a first-cut approach to addressing this issue. More detailed analyses should be completed that segment the population by income level, personal wealth, and health status to get a better understanding of the potential market for LHCP customers. In addition, the critical assumptions discussed at the end of the chapter should be taken into consideration as more detailed reviews are completed.

A FINANCIAL PLANNER'S PERSPECTIVE

Financial planners offer a number of approaches for personal budgeting. These rules typically change over time and will be a function of each person's investment goals and their level of income. Looking at these rules through a broad-brush approach can give some insights into how much Americans are advised to dedicate to health care spending and personal savings today.

One rule of thumb is the 50/30/20 rule. Half of one's after-tax income should go to fixed payments, like mortgages and car payments. Another 30% should go to flexible spending, like groceries and entertainment. The final 20% should be spent on savings and debt payments (student loan, credit card). These are broad categories, and personal health care spending might be included in fixed payments (for health insurance premiums) and flex spending (for over-the-counter and noncovered health care services).

Other estimates suggest that 25% to 35% of after-tax income should be spent on the home (mortgage payments, utilities); 15% to 20% on savings; 10% on groceries; 10% on entertainment; 5% to 10% on transportation; 5% to 10% on debt payments; 5% to 10% on personal health care expenses (health insurance premiums, co-pays, deductible costs); and the remainder (if there is any!) on charitable giving or other miscellaneous categories.

The 5% to 10% estimate of after-tax income for personal health care expenses seems to be an accepted industry standard, at least for those who are non-elderly. The Kaiser Family Foundation estimates that the average annual premium cost for a single (nonfamily) American for 2017 was $6,690. The average American paid 18% of that cost, or $1,204. That means the employer paid the balance, or $5,486.[1] Today, the $1,204 payment, as well as other payments related to health care costs (deductibles, co-pays, out-of-pocket expenses) would come out of the 5% to 10% of after-tax income that individuals should budget for personal health care expenses. (Note that many employees contract for their family's insurance through their employer. Their monthly premiums would be higher than the $1,204 premium shown.

I am using the individual, single plan payment because I am comparing one person's contributions to the health care system to the average *per person* [per capita] costs for health care in America.)

The 5% to 10% budget range should probably be much higher for some individuals who do not have employer-sponsored health insurance. However, at least in 2017 and through 2018, the majority of individuals buying health insurance on the exchange (meaning they didn't get it from their employer) received subsidies for their premium payments. As noted earlier, this group represents less than 10% of the total population. *For this analysis I will use data for individuals with single (not family) plans who receive insurance from their employer.*

The elderly, despite being covered by Medicare and because they are advanced in age, pay a higher percentage of their income on health care. On average, a median-income senior citizen will pay about 20% of their retirement income on health care expenses.[2]

In the Dream Plan, the dollar equivalent of the 20% of retirement income that seniors pay for health care should come from their LHCP, not from their retirement savings account. Therefore, the money that Americans save for retirement today would be split into two separate categories. About 80% of the dollars would go toward a traditional retirement fund. The other 20% would go into an LHCP. In my analysis, I will assume that 20% of the 15% to 20% that should be allocated to savings in today's recommended approach to financial planning will go to the LHCP. *This equates to about 3% to 4% in after-tax income that will be directed to an LHCP to be saved for health care expenses.*

Americans contribute much more to overall health care expenditures because a portion of the dollars does not come out of their household budgets. Identifying these categories helps provide a more comprehensive perspective on how much is paid into the health care system by individuals or on behalf of individuals.

TAXES AND OTHER CONTRIBUTIONS

First come taxes. The gross (before tax) income of working Americans is subject to a 1.45% payroll tax for Medicare. This figure went up for some Americans after ACA was passed. Individuals earning over $200,000 a year became subject to the Additional Medicare Tax.[3] Any income over $200,000 is taxed at 2.35%, or the base 1.45%—plus an extra 0.9%. High earners may also be hit with the Net Investment Income Tax (NIIT).[4] This is a 3.8% tax targeted at investment income (not payroll) at certain levels over regular income. *In my model, the average American only pays 1.45% for the Medicare payroll tax.*

As outlined in chapter 2, Medicare is funded not just through payroll taxes, but also through sources including contributions from different types of taxes collected by the federal government and distributions from the Medicare Trust Fund. Federal and state governments also collect taxes, and then these dollars are reallocated to different budgetary priorities that include Medicare and Medicaid (as well as other categories like education, infrastructure, and state employee retirement payments). A forensic financial expert could have a field day trying to map how an individual's taxes get routed through the system to pay for the Medicare and Medicaid public health programs. As far as this high-level analysis is concerned, I will not try to estimate these indirect contributions. Instead, *I will assume that whatever is collected and allocated through indirect payments will not be saved by the individual in an LHCP but will go toward funding public health.* However, as noted previously, I will assume that the 1.45% that the individual directly pays for the Medicare payroll tax would become a contribution to an LHCP.

Employers, on behalf of their employees, contribute a significant chunk of health care dollars, too. First, they match the 1.45% Medicare payroll tax that their employees pay, and send that to Uncle Sam. (They're not responsible for the high-income surcharge, however.)

Most employers also pay for a portion of their employees' health insurance, about two-thirds (for family) or more (for single) of the cost for the average premium. In our example, the employer pays 82% of the annual premium payment, or $5,486, while an employee contributes $1,204. Employers may also subsidize other perks such as gym memberships and on-site wellness clinics. Employees are not taxed on these benefits, which is a bone of contention for many people, including me.[5]

While these dollars are not paid directly to the individual, they can be attributed to the individual. In an LHCP environment, these dollars should be redirected to the individual as cash payments or employer contributions to an LHCP. In such a scenario, they would be considered income and would be subject to tax. But in terms of my model, I am trying to determine whether the dollars contributed in the system today by individuals or on behalf of individuals could cover the annual per capita cost of care. *Therefore, my model will allocate the entire $5,486 as a contribution to the LHCP from the employer.*

Redirecting the Medicare payroll tax paid by the employer into an LHCP is a different story. While the tax paid by the employer is based on the income of the employee, Medicare is not reserving those dollars for that employee to use at a later date. The money is used by Medicare to fund the payments for current Medicare beneficiaries and to support the program's other initiatives and requirements. The payment is related to the employee but can't be attributed to the employee because the employee doesn't glean any benefit from the payment in the current year. *Therefore, I will exclude the Medicare payroll tax paid by the employer from the analysis.*

MAKING THE COMPARISON

As noted in the LHCP Business Case Detail, the average American's contributions to the health care system today that could be contributed to an LHCP is $10,396 (line14). This figure approximates the average annual health care expenditures per capita for 2017, or $10,745 (line 18). The difference between these two figures is a little over 3%. The model does not include indirect contributions that Americans make through other taxes that I assumed would go toward funding public health. If those contributions were estimated, they would increase the

$10,396 figure, potentially bringing it more in line with the $10,745, or the estimated per capita costs for health care for 2017.

Americans should feel confident that the LHCP model could work, given some critical assumptions.

CRITICAL ASSUMPTIONS

ACCESS TO EMPLOYER CONTRIBUTIONS

The wiggliest expectation is that employees would gain access to the full financial contributions their employers make to their health care premiums today. The LHCP's reliance on these payments demonstrates the outsized role that employers currently have on subsidizing health care costs in America. It also highlights a huge gap in the affordability of health care between those who do and do not receive employer-sponsored contributions.

In the Dream Plan, private insurance would not exist. Yet employers may still want to provide—and more importantly, employees may still expect to receive—a contribution toward employee health care costs. If employers do offer such a contribution, the individual would likely receive it as a cash payment, potentially akin to a 401(k)-matching contribution. The money would either be taxed as income when it gets distributed to the employee, there may be some income tax deferral benefit assigned to the payment, or it may be taxed some other way. But it will probably be taxed. That means the amount that would come across in my model would be lower by whatever effective tax rate applies to the payment.

Assuming the funds are invested in an LHCP, they would grow significantly over a period of decades. This would give individuals with access to employer-sponsored payments in the Dream Plan even more of an advantage over those who do not receive them today. Right now, the benefit employees receive from getting subsidized care is basically an avoidance of payment, or a pass-through from the employer to the insurance company. In the Dream Plan, if employees receive this money in cash to be invested, they'll get the benefit of having their health care costs subsidized (the pass-through) and they'll also benefit by collecting the additional income earned by investing it.

Of course, employers may balk at making the payments altogether. I am sure many employers would love to eliminate their employee-sponsored health insurance payments. My guess is that some employers would offer some sort of benefit while others would not, and overall, employees would receive less money for health care from their employers than they do today.

LHCP PLAN HOLDERS WILL
HAVE FINANCIAL DISCIPLINE

The typical American does not do a very good job of saving for retirement. Baby boomers have a median retirement savings of $147,000. Gen X folks have saved about $69,000 for retirement, while Millennials have about $31,000 put away.[6] All estimates indicate that these figures will not provide these individuals with the income they'll need to live comfortable lives in retirement. Since we're not savers now, it's difficult to expect that most Americans will have the discipline to save money for a new kind of investment product like an LHCP.

Individuals with higher levels of income are more likely to save because they can cover their basic living costs and still put money aside for future use. High-income individuals are more likely to be early adapters in the LHCP because they'll have the money to abide by the program's requirements.

An essential component of gaining more and more LHCP enrollees will be to help them find ways to save money. The most effective method is to direct payments from an employee's payroll into their LHCP accounts. This will result in a dramatic drop in income for many employees. Bracing for a change in both spending and savings will be a critical success factor for the adoption of LHCPs.

Today, money in investment accounts, like 401(k)s, can be withdrawn before the recommended investment time period has been achieved. Individuals in financial hardship may liquidate all or part of their 401(k) accounts, expecting to save money later for their retirement. Many of them don't. As a result, they may find themselves in a tenuous financial position later in life. Such behavior must be prohibited in the Dream Plan. An individual's ability to access the money in an LHCP for anything else except health care expenses must be severely restricted. Otherwise, they won't have the money they'll need when they'll need it the most.

HEALTH CARE COSTS SHOULDN'T BE SO HIGH

My analysis shows that the amount of money paid for or associated with an individual today approximates the average health care costs per person in America. A key issue with the analysis is that the largest line item, the employer contribution, will flow completely to the employee when the Dream Plan is rolled out. With the elimination of employer-sponsored health care in the Dream Plan, employees are likely to see a reduction in this benefit. Then their health care savings would not cover the current health care costs per capita.

But using the current health care costs per capita as a bogey for savings assumes that our current cost structure for health care is acceptable. It isn't. It should be much lower. How do we get there?

CHAPTER 11

HOW THE DREAM PLAN CAN REDUCE COSTS IN HEALTH CARE

Any proposal to transform the health care system must result in a significant reduction of costs. In this chapter, I will discuss several ways the Dream Plan concepts can pull costs out of the system.

LHCP COMPANIES ASK QUESTIONS TODAY'S INSURERS CAN'T

From the perspective of a health insurer, risk relates to the unknown health care needs that an enrollee of their program might require at any given time. Insurers, whether offering ACA plans or employer-sponsored products, use detailed analytics to project what they believe the expenses for a given group will be. Yet there is always the risk that these projections may be incorrect and/or that unexpected events might impact the financial needs of a member pool. To shield against this, insurers charge a premium on rates above the actual projected cost of care.

As part of the Affordable Care Act, insurers offering marketplace plans are prohibited from discriminating against potential enrollees due to preexisting conditions, and they do not ask for family histories. Insurers don't know if an applicant has a family history of breast cancer, if they've recently been diagnosed with fibromyalgia (pain, fatigue, and an inability to concentrate), or if they've been suffering from depression for the past ten years. Even many employer-sponsored health plans are hampered in their ability to mitigate risk due to limited access to information resulting from factors such as a company's human resources policy and regulations related to employee privacy and data security. As a result, current insurance models have a significant amount of unnecessary risk built into their pricing. Prices are higher than they need to be because insurers cannot get an accurate profile of the individuals who sign up for their plans.

The LHCP eliminates a significant amount of this risk because plan designers can ask enrollees all the questions that today's insurance companies can't. Genetic testing, historical health information, and family histories are key inputs into identifying an individual's projected health needs.

And the LHCP goes even further in mitigating risk because it collects more information that traditional insurers do. Genetics and family history information are static data points and don't change over time. Yet an individual's behavior is likely to shift considerably. These behavioral modifications will have dramatic influence over an individual's proclivity to develop the diseases identified in a genetic test or family history. The LHCP can also identify whether externalities, such as living in a community with a high concentration of lead in the water or the long-term stress of a high-powered job, can predict the onset of serious disease or dangerous episodic events.

When so many unknowns are eliminated, a significant amount of risk is reduced. When risk is reduced, costs should also come down.

Look at it this way: Why insure yourself against developing cancer when all your risk factors indicate that you're not going to get it?

GETTING RID OF OVERDESIGNED HEALTH PLANS

The Dream Plan also improves upon conventional insurance by "right-sizing" the insurance options in each LHCP, based on individual preferences. This customization is the inverse of the one-size-fits-all, comprehensive health plan coverage options that Americans have gotten used to. Now, health insurance is likely to cover primary care, emergency services, inpatient and outpatient care, rehabilitation, mental health services, and a variety of drugs.

Yet these generous plans are sometimes problematic because they can incent overutilization. Low co-pays and generous drug coverage encourage unnecessary use because enrollees don't pay much, if anything, out of pocket to access these benefits. Individuals consider these benefits "free" despite the fact that the cost of using them is built into their health plans. They may access these services, like making multiple appointments with a primary care doctor or specialist for minor problems that could clear up in a day, or for follow-ups that are unnecessary. Physicians may order medications that the enrollee has no intention of taking, but the patient fills the prescriptions anyway because the co-pay is low or is zero. These sorts of behaviors bloat costs without necessarily improving outcomes.

The ACA attempted to ratchet back the costs in these generous employer-based plans through the so-called Cadillac Tax. A 40% tax on a portion of the cost for high-dollar employer-sponsored plans was supposed to go into effect in 2018 but has been pushed out to 2022. Employers don't want to pay the taxes, employees don't want the taxes passed through to them, and insurers want to make sure that employers continue to contract for the benefits. As a result, these high costs will remain in the system until the Cadillac Tax takes effect—should that day ever come.

While attempting to curb the excesses of some employer-sponsored plans with the Cadillac Tax, the ACA, ironically, mandated the enhancement of offerings in other health insurance plans. As I have discussed previously, any plan offered through the health care exchanges was required to include coverage for ten essential benefits. Some customers had no choice but to buy plans that included services they didn't want or wouldn't use.

The Dream Plan addresses these problems because every LHCP is customized for the individual. Customers will budget for the health care services they're projected to need in a care plan designed exclusively for them. Because they'll be spending their own money directly, they'll be encouraged to find the right doctors and get the most out of their visits so they're not paying more than they need to. They'll use the therapies and drugs that are most effective to address their conditions. They may question the necessity of certain procedures and what may seem like excessive tests.

Importantly, LHCP members will need to be counseled against care avoidance as a means to save money when the prescribed care is medically beneficial. It's one thing to skip a follow-up appointment with a dermatologist if that rash you've been complaining about has resolved itself and disappeared. It's an entirely different case to skip a preventive colonoscopy. Customers must remember that the frequency and types of care in the LHCP have been designed specifically for them. Cutting corners in the short term can create negative health outcomes in the long term.

LONGITUDINAL PERSPECTIVE

The LHCP creates a budget for an individual's lifetime health care costs. It estimates the dollars that will be needed over the decades of an individual's life. This differs from how health care is managed today. Right now, both public and private insurers work around budgets for set time periods, almost always using a twelve-month time frame to monitor key financial and operational metrics. Customers enrolling in insurance plans are also impacted by this annual horizon. Each year, individuals must renew or buy new insurance. Deductibles are reset to zero after twelve months. This short-term perspective creates misaligned incentives in today's health care system that can be eliminated in the Dream Plan.

SWITCHING COSTS

Every time an individual switches their insurance, administrative and even some medical costs are incurred. Insurers spend money on advertising and other promotional efforts to attract customers. When an individual switches plans, the new company expends administrative resources to enroll them. All these activities add costs to the system.

From a clinical perspective, switching insurers means that patients may have to switch doctors. If their current doctor is not contracted with their new insurer, the physician with the new plan may need to rechart that patient's medical history. As discussed, there is little interoperability in the health care system. That makes it hard for a new doctor to access a patient's old records. In many cases, they'll simply reorder tests and rerun bloodwork to get the current information they need about a patient.

Switching insurance contributes to the health care system's already problematic concerns over data fragmentation. Patient information winds up in the hands of multiple insurance companies and multiple providers. This dispersion of data increases the potential for the exposure of personal health information through data breaches.

INABILITY TO REASONABLY COMPARE PLANS

Ironically, many individuals think that competition in the health insurance market is good for consumers. Each year buyers are encouraged to log on to healthcare.gov and compare plans so they can get the best deal. Choice is also offered through employer-based plans, as many large employers offer their employees insurance from more than one carrier.

Yet many individuals do not have a clear understanding of all the terms and conditions of the health insurance products they're comparing. The key criteria that consumers use when selecting a health plan are the monthly premium, the deductible, and whether their preferred doctor is part of the plan. Few people scrutinize the particular services offered, and even fewer drill down to the point where they can use the number of covered services as a differentiating factor between plans.

For example, some plans may cover four primary care visits a year, while another may only cover two. One plan may cover twelve rehabilitation sessions with a physical therapist, and another will only cover eight. How is an individual supposed to know not only which services they want but also how many of them they're going to need?

Insurers might argue that they're giving customers "choice" by offering plans with varying levels of coverage related to both the services offered and the volume of services covered. Those who go to the doctor frequently may choose plans with more visits covered. Those who are expecting to have surgery, such as a planned hip replacement, may opt for a plan with more coverage for physical therapy.

Unfortunately, the plans don't provide line-item or menu-type pricing. In other words, a customer can't determine how much more they should be spending just to get the extra primary care visits or physical therapy sessions because costs for so many options are summed up together. The variability in plan offerings creates unnecessary complexity and drives up costs in the system.

THE FALLACY OF INTERSTATE HEALTH PLAN BENEFITS

Offering insurance across state lines is also an ineffective means to reduce costs in the health care system. Proponents of interstate health plan shopping may not appreciate the complexity associated with providing services in local markets, especially in different states. The complexity is driven by the fact that offering health insurance requires insurers to not only set rates for services, but also to contract with individuals and organizations to provide those services.

For example, an insurer in Kentucky that wants to offer insurance in West Virginia would need familiarity with the local markets in that state. The difficulty of getting the necessary information would be compounded by the fact that plans would have to satisfy the ACA's ten essential benefits burden. So, the insurer isn't just looking for a hospital and big physician practice so they can offer insurance. They'll also need relationships with mental health professionals, rehab providers, and others. Further, the insurer would have to understand the impact of any state-specific regulations, which can drive up the cost of contracting. Who pays for those higher costs? Consumers.

In addition, interstate insurance plans favor large companies over small businesses. The top insurance companies in America already offer plans in multiple states. But many small, regional insurers lack the expertise to develop the contractual arrangements they'll need to offer plans in other states. As a result, a regionally based company may fall victim to a price war with a national company. The national insurer may sacrifice the profitability of plans offered in the same markets served by the small company by lowering its rates to the point that the smaller company's customers switch over. That can drive the small insurer out of business. Such action enables the larger company to drive up rates later, when competition has been eliminated.

PRICE/QUALITY CONUNDRUM

Today's health insurance models make it hard to prioritize a patient's longitudinal health benefits over a health plan's short-term budgetary restrictions. Many insurers, including Medicare and Medicaid, do not allow providers free rein in prescribing care options that may have the most impactful longitudinal benefits for patients. Instead, insurers dictate specific allowable options—from the drugs they can prescribe to the types of medical devices they are permitted to use in a procedure. Providers must make trade-offs between the costs of these allowable options and the quality of the outcomes that can be generated.

Oftentimes, plans, both public and private, will only allow for inexpensive health care goods and services with the intent of providing coverage to more beneficiaries. The problem arises when the rate that the insurer will pay for a good (like a drug) or service (like a doctor's time) is so low that it results in low-quality care. This is a key problem with Medicaid. Some doctors simply refuse to see Medicaid patients for a number of reasons, one of which is that the reimbursement from CMS is lower than what other insurers typically pay. As a result, Medicaid patients have fewer options for care. They are excluded from access to some high-quality doctors simply because these doctors will not participate in the program. Such an exclusion lowers the quality of care that Medicaid enrollees receive.

The price/quality conundrum also applies to products. A good example relates to implants used in joint replacement surgery. Some implants are more expensive, but they are more durable, made of better materials, and/or may be better designed to meet the specific needs of the patient. These higher-cost options can increase the mobility of the patient, improving their quality of life and their ability to work or even live independently. The implant may never need to be replaced, enabling the patient to avoid the hardship of an additional surgery later in life, as well as eliminating the expense of the second procedure. All of these factors improve outcomes and reduce not only costs in the health care system, but dollars spent on social services and family resources, impacting the economy as a whole.

If that higher-priced, higher-quality implant is not approved by the insurer, the patient is unlikely to receive it. It's a trade-off many insurers are willing to make. Private insurers are inclined to use cheaper options because the likelihood is low that a patient will be part of the insurer's program by the time the longitudinal impacts of the low-quality implant manifest themselves. The patient may switch to another insurer. If the patient is close to qualifying for Medicare, there's even less of an incentive to give them a high-quality implant because the government will be responsible for paying for the individual's health care costs in just a few years.

The longitudinal management of an individual's health care is an essential factor in the LHCP's effectiveness. Individuals are encouraged to establish a strong, long-term relationship with a provider of choice, which is made easier because they are not restricted by an insurer's programmatic requirements. Since patients are, basically, self-insured, they avoid all the pitfalls presented from a lifetime of swapping insurance coverage. And since they're spending their own money, they can make the cost and quality trade-offs for care based on their preferences and their budget.

SELF-SUFFICIENCY AND SELF-RATIONING

One of the quintessential American Dream ideologies is self-sufficiency. Self-sufficiency implies that each of us is in control. When we're in control, we have choice, we have options. The LHCP gives Americans the choice and the options they need to create a health plan that matches their needs. But in many cases, the choice some Americans will have to make is not between one thing and another; it will be between *having* one thing and *not having* one thing. In order to be self-sufficient with regard to funding our own health care, many of us will need to self-ration.

The spending philosophy for any American enrolled in an LHCP is that the care they design should be within the parameters they can afford. This philosophy shifts some of the responsibility for correcting America's problem with overutilization to the average American— away from the physician and away from the government.

MEDICAL PROFESSIONALS MUST HELP RATION CARE

Of course, individuals do not have the expertise to develop a lifelong health care plan on their own. As discussed, customers will work with medical professionals and LHCP financial advisers to balance the resources they have with the health care they're expected to need.

As part of this rationing exercise, an individual's personal preferences must be balanced with the medical community's recommended protocols for care. If an individual is projected to develop cancer, the rationing process should not exclude the cost of the typical treatment for the cancer, which may be surgery and chemotherapy. Individuals will not be encouraged to give up medications to treat their HIV in lieu of alternative, naturopathic concoctions. Foregoing proven, albeit expensive treatment options may only make individuals sicker, less able to contribute to society, and ultimately more of a burden to their communities.

USING BEHAVIORAL MODIFICATIONS TO RATION CARE

The notion of rationing implies that resources are somehow constrained. An individual is up against a resource constraint if they need more care than they can afford. This situation can be addressed in one of two ways.

Individuals may seek to increase their income. In other words, they may look for higher-paying employment or take on a second job to improve their financial position to the point that they can afford the care they've designed. These are viable options for some people, but not all Americans will have the opportunity or the drive or the capability to dramatically increase their income. As a result, if they want to have an LHCP, they'll need to find a way to lower their health care costs.

The simplest approach to doing so is to forego components in an individual's LHCP that are not essential to achieving one's health care goals. As discussed earlier, individuals may reduce the frequency of certain encounters, like chiropractic visits or massage therapy. They can switch to using generic drugs and store-branded products, which are cheaper and oftentimes provide the same level of quality as brand-name goods. These are some examples of incremental changes that can be undertaken to make an individual's health care budget more affordable.

A more consequential approach to self-rationing is to focus not on limiting treatment options, but on eliminating disease. The LHCP provides customers with the ability to see into the future. They'll know the diseases they are projected to develop. If these diseases are in any way preventable, then customers should be incented to modify their behavior to forestall or eliminate their manifestation—and avoid the costs to treat them.

This approach to "demand reduction" may be one of the most important aspects of the Dream Plan. The LHCP will enable self-sufficiency through a self-rationing process that incents Americans to improve their health so they can afford the care they want.

BOTH HEALTH AND WEALTH AFFECT SELF-RATIONING

This delicate self-rationing exercise will be impacted by two factors: relative wealth and health. As outlined below, those with considerable wealth will have less of a need, if any, to self-ration. Those with few resources and significant health demands will be more incented to self-ration or they will qualify for the public health program.

CHART 12. FACTORS IMPACTING SELF-RATIONING

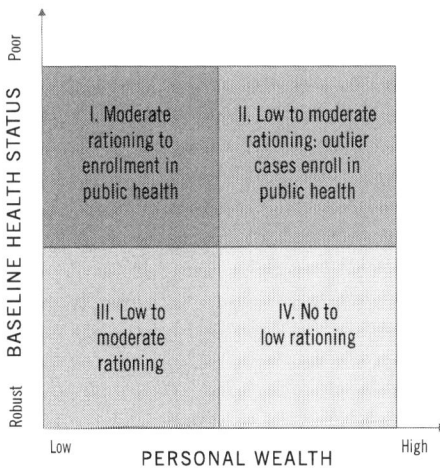

Those with considerable personal wealth (Quadrants II and IV) will have access to the care they want, regardless of their health requirements. The very wealthy might still be able to afford the care necessary for individuals impacted with debilitating issues. Less wealthy individuals may be able to afford their own care by rationing some non-essential needs or by using crowdfunding platforms to enhance their LHCP investment.

An interesting aspect of the Dream Plan is that it elevates the importance of health status as a means to provide individuals with more control over the health care they can access. Today, individuals with low personal wealth are either uninsured or qualify for Medicaid (and Medicare, depending on their age). As discussed earlier, individuals on Medicaid have, on average, fewer choices and access to lower-quality health care. That makes their ability to improve their health status more difficult than it should be.

There are poor Americans who are in good health. And there are low-income Americans who would respond to a system that rewards them with the freedom of choice if they are able to maintain a healthy life. These individuals would fall into Quadrant III in the graphic. They'd be able to have their own LHCP because their health profile was such that they would be able to afford the care they'd require.

Liberating this group from the public health pool is a win for all Americans. First, these individuals can be more empowered and will be encouraged to lead healthier, happier, more productive lives. Taxpayers will also be less burdened with funding the care for these individuals, as they will be able to take care of themselves. And the public health program itself will be smaller, making it easier to more effectively manage.

Individuals with low income and considerable health concerns will fall into Quadrant I. Some may be able to ration to a point where they can still provide for themselves, but many may default into a public health program. As will be discussed in the next chapter, individuals who are on public health programs would still be required to contribute part of their income to the pool to fund services.

PLANNING FOR DEATH

Health care expenses spike as individuals advance in age. As discussed in the Introduction, many Americans do not prepare themselves for the emotional and medical decisions that will have to be made related to their care when they're older. Here's a disturbing fact: One in three senior citizens dies with Alzheimer's or dementia.[1] That means that many of us will not have the intellectual capacity to make informed health care decisions for ourselves when we're older. We all need to plan for death.

Planning for death isn't just necessary for those who may develop cognitive deficiencies. Every LHCP customer will have established a philosophy about the kind of health care they want, and they will have budgeted for the services that support their plan. For example, those who prefer a homeopathic approach to health care may have a limited budget for prescription medication. These individuals are probably low utilizers of care and may not want to access complicated surgeries and myriad drug combinations to address their illnesses as they age. Risk-averse individuals may budget for extra tests and second opinions when making consequential health care choices. These folks may be more conservative when given ranges of outcomes and might opt for aggressive surgery to address a potential condition rather than a wait-and-see option.

As individuals age, they may change their mind about how they want their health care administered. If they haven't saved enough money to fund these shifts in preferences, they may expect the financial burden for their care to be carried by others. This situation must be managed proactively to ensure that we all remain self-sufficient through the last days of our lives.

Consider an eighty-nine-year-old man whose personal philosophy is to maintain wellness as a means to avoid nonessential drugs and unnecessary treatments. He's lived a good life. His late-in-life plan is to reject medical care for debilitating, life-threatening conditions. If he gets cancer, which his LHCP has predicted will come, his plan is to die with dignity rather than undergo painful, expensive surgery or chemotherapy that may not even save him.

Right before his ninetieth birthday, his wife of almost seventy years dies suddenly of pneumonia. He is destitute. He's lonely and he becomes petrified of dying. He tells his children to rip up his do not resuscitate (DNR) order. In other words, if he becomes medically incapacitated (like if his heart stops from a heart attack), he now wants the medical community to try to bring him back to life. This is a total reversal of his death plan.

Sure enough, several days later, he has a stroke. Doctors try to revive him, but they can't bring him back to full consciousness. He winds up in a vegetative state on life support. Doctors say he has almost no chance of ever waking up.

Who's supposed to pay for his care?

With a depleted LHCP, the cost for this patient's care shouldn't become the burden of the public health system. The cost of his care could divert millions of dollars from the necessary treatments needed by other Americans. The government may be pressured to act in a manner that some may consider humane, at the cost of either redirecting funds from others or simply going over budget.

But there is hope.

As discussed earlier, coordination among charity groups and donors should be improved under the Dream Plan. Just as some individuals may wish to fund a drug annuity program for HIV-AIDS patients (as described in chapter 9), others may wish to contribute funds for patients on life support. Finding creative ways to address the variety of values and needs in our culture—as opposed to developing one system that tries to address them all—will be a critical element of ensuring that Americans can live and die as they wish.

CHAPTER 12

PUBLIC HEALTH

The Dream Plan calls for two options for health coverage: an LHCP and public health. Any American who possesses the financial resources to fund their own care would have an LHCP. All others would qualify for a public health program. In this section, I will consider public health as it might be designed, given the two-option scenario.

DETERMINING WHO QUALIFIES FOR PUBLIC HEALTH

LHCP customers partner with physicians to plan for the health care they want within the budgets they can afford. The hard part is defining "within the budgets they can afford" because that definition is the dividing linc between those who qualify for an LCHP and those who will enroll in public health.

I believe this dividing line will be determined over time by Americans as more and more people enroll in LHCPs. Government officials will be able to understand how typical LHCP holders budget for their own health care. These models can then be used as benchmarks to help develop budgets for individuals enrolled in public health. It will take time for the LHCP market to mature so that this data can be used effectively.

Early adapters of the LHCP model will probably be wealthier and healthier than the average American. These individuals would be in a reasonable position to accept the risk of enrolling in a new and unproven product. Their LHCPs may have more health care services than may be necessary, because they may not ration care. At this point, it would be too soon to use the LHCPs that have been created as models for public health because none of the participants in the program would have been particularly price sensitive.

As the LHCP becomes a more proven product, it will be less risky to the general public. Those with fewer resources are more likely to participate. These individuals may be in better than average health, which lowers their financial exposure and further reduces their risk in participating. Nonetheless, they will add more dimensions to the data set, allowing further insights into preferred and more effective protocols for care.

Some enrollees may be very sick. These individuals may be more likely to ration some care. Their approach to structuring an LHCP can provide significant insights for public health officials about the effectiveness of different approaches to health care for the very ill.

As time goes by, LHCP companies will start to identify preferred care protocols for its customers. New LHCP customers may be offered a baseline care protocol that's tailored to them once their genetic testing and background information have been analyzed. This can help make the initial design of the LHCP less expensive because customers can customize a "straw man" rather than create a product from scratch. Public health officials may also access this information to help them design their programs.

At some point, the market should reach an equilibrium where a certain standard of care protocols will be identified for individuals with different genetic, behavioral, and income profiles. The determination of whether individuals should be able to afford an LHCP will be derived from the most democratic of mechanisms: crowdsourcing.

THE DREAM PLAN DEMOCRATIZES PUBLIC HEALTH CARE

Public health programs struggle to provide the right type and amount of care to the constituents it serves for the amount of money it's been given to spend. I've criticized the Medicaid and Medicare programs a lot in this book because the outcomes they've produced should be a whole lot better than they are. But that doesn't mean that running CMS, or any other public health program, is easy. There's always a new drug on the market, there's always a group lobbying for more care, and the political ramifications of restricting access to care are a political nightmare for elected officials. It's hard for public health officials to resist these pressures and stay on budget.

Fortunately, the Dream Plan provides a solution to this problem. Public health officials can use the care protocols identified in LHCPs as guidelines to create their budgets. Imagine a time when LHCPs have become mainstream in America. Consolidating the information in all the LHCPs would provide a powerful data set for government officials (and anyone else who'd want to study it). It would contain the care preferences of individuals as determined *by the people* (in collaboration with their medical professionals, of course).

In other words, officials could look at all the LHCPs of, say, a female with a certain set of genetic characteristics, living in an urban environment, who smokes and is divorced with two children. Given that profile (and more likely, one that incorporates many more factors), public health officials could budget the same amount of money for the enrollees in public health that customers with a similar background who had LHCPs spent on themselves.

Such a scenario democratizes health care by putting everyone on a more level playing field. Public health officials could be somewhat shielded from complaints about the second-class care that the poor and needy receive because they'd be using the same care protocols as everyone else. Further, advocates for this constituency would have a hard time lobbying for even more care than what's been budgeted for the poor. If the average American isn't willing to pay for more care than what has been identified in their self-funded LHCP, then those on public health, who are relying on payments from others, shouldn't have more generous access to it.

Some may argue that the care required by average LHCP customers is insufficient to address the needs of the poor. As noted, income is a major external determinant of health, and those with low incomes have, typically, lower outcomes. The Dream Plan seeks to address this problem through health education and wellness promotion. As discussed, annual primary care visits are required to provide individuals with the education they need to improve their health. Education and better physician/patient partnerships should help reduce the substandard outcomes associated with lower-income Americans.

The Dream Plan assumes that providers will be paid directly by patients (if they have an LHCP) or on behalf of patients (if they're on public health). Providers will establish one rate for services, implying that the government will not reimburse at a lower-than-market rate. Such an approach should improve the quality of care that low-income individuals receive because they'd have access to the same doctors, drugs, programs, etc. that would be used by the average American.

EVERYTHING COMES WITH A COST

Public health officials and the American public are going to have to determine whether individuals enrolled in public health will have their own publicly funded LHCP, or whether public health officials will be given the discretion to spend the money associated with the care identified in an average American's LHCP plan on their own. There are pros and cons associated with each scenario.

Given the complexity of creating an LHCP, public health officials are likely to contract with private sector companies who have established expertise and demonstrated success. That service will come at a cost. Governmental agencies may wish to develop their own LHCPs at some point too. Regardless of who operates the program, certain functionality will be required.

Unfortunately, the upside of expending all these resources might not outweigh the costs. An LHCP is most effective if the individual is motivated to manage their health. Many LHCP customers are incented to improve their health because they're paying for the care themselves. Public health enrollees don't have such an incentive. They won't save money if they improve their health.

Therefore, the health system must continue to make efforts to incent the public health constituency to improve its health simply for the sheer benefit of being in good health. Our current system has been ineffective at providing the poor with the tools and motivation that many of them need to help themselves. The Dream Plan seeks to address this problem through better education and coordination with caregivers. But some individuals may simply not go to the doctor. They may not be interested in accurately completing their externalities assessment. They may fail to report for consultative sessions. As a result, the data set available to LHCP operators will be insufficient to generate relevant projections. The LHCP simply won't work.

RATIONING

The Dream Plan requires that public health officials spend only the amount of funding that's been budgeted for their programs. Using the dollars associated in average Americans' LHCPs provides these administrators with a fair estimation of the amount of resources that should be expended on enrollees in public health.

Let's assume that the allocated dollars are aggregated into one lump sum that will be divvied up among the members of the public health pool. The same stressors that cause public health programs to overspend today could very well impact public health officials tomorrow—even though they've been provided with a good estimation of the amount of dollars required to deliver care.

One challenge is that the dollars provided to public officials would be based on averages. Most individuals will not be "average." Some will require more care, and others will require less. It will be up to the officials to make sure that those who require more care don't receive an outsized portion of the funding. In order to stay on budget, officials will need to ration some of the dollars.

Importantly, we should be reminded that many Americans with LHCPs will be self-rationing to ensure that they can afford their care. In other words, rationing won't just be for those on public health.

Rationing is a controversial topic. The concept conjures images of sterile meeting rooms with white-coated surveyors impassively using statistics to make life-and-death situations. Yet rationing can be a positive exercise. It should be viewed as a disciplined mechanism to optimize care distribution among the public health population.

Lessons can be learned from countries that ration health care services, including Canada and the United Kingdom. Typically, most public health programs allow certain basic services to be covered. Review boards are in place to determine whether selected high-cost drugs, surgeries, and/or therapies will be approved for different individuals. Similar boards should be created in public health for the Dream Plan.

Using health metrics as a means to ration care may also be an option. This concept has been floated with considerable controversy by the UK's National Health Service (NHS). In late 2017, NHS proposed an indefinite delay on nonelective surgeries for smokers or those who are overweight.[1] The proposal would require individuals to stop smoking for eight weeks and/or lose weight in order to qualify for selected operations.

This approach to care rationing has its challenges. First off, it's difficult to determine whether an individual has abided by the non-smoking requirement. Doing so might require monitoring the nicotine levels in the enrollee's blood. Capturing this information is costly. Some may argue that doing so violates an individual's privacy and civil rights. As for the weight loss condition, the obese may object due to the fact that they *need* the elective surgery in order to help them lose weight. Their circular protest would be that they can't qualify for the surgery because they need the surgery to help them qualify for the surgery.

Fortunately, there are mechanisms that could be deployed to help ration care in the public health arena.

REQUIREMENTS OF PUBLIC HEALTH ENROLLEES

First and foremost, every American should be required to see their primary care doctor every year. Annual checkups can provide wonderful trend information and data tracking for the preventive care needs of public health enrollees. Preventive screenings and education are critical components to improving health and reducing overall costs in the system.

Individuals will default into public health if the dollars they earn can't cover their estimated health care costs. Such automatic enrollment could incent some individuals to not work at all. Yet everyone whose care is funded by public health programs should contribute to society at a level commensurate with their capabilities and interest. They should either work or satisfy the requirement by volunteering with an array of governmentally approved organizations. In some cases these requirements may be waived for the infirm, for pregnant women, and for guardians of young children with no access to child care. Worker requirements for Medicaid have already begun to gain traction in some states today.[2]

In the Dream Plan, individuals who do not visit a PCP or do not complete their work/volunteer contributions would be penalized through a rationing process. All factors being equal, preference for a drug or service should be given to an individual who has historically visited a primary care doctor and completed their work requirements over someone who has not. This is an approach to care access that promotes wellness and encourages all Americans to be active contributors to society.

PUBLIC ENROLLEES' FINANCIAL CONTRIBUTIONS

Using income as a qualification metric for access to public health can disincentivize certain individuals from seeking out higher-paying jobs. Those whose incomes are close to but just under the qualification limits may lose money if they make more of it because their increase will push them out of the public health pool and require them to pay for their own care. If the cost of their care is more than their income boost, their brand-new job may leave them worse off financially than before.

A key difference between public health programs of today (particularly in comparison to Medicaid) and the Dream Plan is that almost all individuals would be required to commit some of their income to the public health pool. They will not be able to cover all the services that they'll need, but almost everyone can contribute something. Doing so lowers the overall burden for their fellow Americans. In addition, some individuals may be more incented to better manage their health if they recognize that some of their own money is going into the system to pay for it.

At the very least, individuals should be expected to contribute the equivalent of the 1.45% Medicare payroll tax that is collected today.

Ideally, a sliding scale of contribution levels should be used to ensure that those public health beneficiaries who are able to contribute some of their income are required to do so. The challenge with this approach is that today's typical Medicaid enrollee is employed but is barely making ends meet. Requiring these individuals to set aside several percentage points of their income to health care is untenable given the amount of money they make. Many of these enrollees are in part-time jobs, are self-employed, or work for companies that are too small to offer them employer-sponsored health insurance.

An essential takeaway from the analyses in this book relates to the critical role that employer-sponsored health insurance plays in the budgets of everyday Americans. When employers contribute money to their employees' health insurance costs, they are de facto acknowledging that a living wage must provide enough money to cover health care expenses. The vast majority of individuals who do not have access to employer-sponsored health insurance simply don't make enough money to cover the costs of health care. These folks are either on Medicaid or they are receiving subsidies for the purchase of premiums in the ACA marketplaces.

In the Dream Plan, there will be no more traditional health insurance. Employers may wish to eliminate all the costs associated with paying for their employees' health care and just reabsorb the dollars into the company business. If they do, they will effectively be cutting compensation to their employees. No doubt such action would meet with both public and governmental resistance. Employers should brace for the need to transfer some of the money that is currently used to subsidize health care costs to their employees (either through salary increases or lump-sum payments or some other mechanism) so employees can afford to buy health care.

Because the intent of the transfer is to ensure that individuals can afford health care, then *all employees* should benefit from the change in policy, not just full-time employees. As a result, lower-income Americans would receive an increase in compensation. That increase could be enough to help some qualify for an LHCP. Others may see the increase pass through to the government in the form of a contribution to health care expenses for individuals enrolled in public health.

As noted earlier, some public health enrollees may be in the program because they have severe health issues. They may have access to sources of income that ordinarily would have kept them out of the public health pool, but their conditions are too expensive to fund on their own. These individuals, like others in public health, should be required to contribute toward their health care needs. One way to establish a payment level would be to use the average rate that LHCP customers of a similar age, sex, and geography pay for their own care. It wouldn't cover all the costs, but it would be a contribution nonetheless.

A targeted outcome of the Dream Plan is a reduction in the number of enrollees in public health, making the program more effective to manage. Many of the ideas proposed in the plan should help improve the health of Americans and drive down the overall cost of care. Doing so should make the cost of health care more affordable to more Americans, enabling more people to enroll in LHCPs.

CHAPTER 13

MAKING OR BREAKING: CRITICAL SUCCESS FACTORS

Companies offering LHCP products will have their work cut out for them. It will take a monumental (but achievable) effort to create a program that safely and securely combines so many disparate data elements to ensure that individuals have enough resources to pay for their health care needs. The critical success factors associated with this movement will be significant and will evolve as the products are embraced by the market.

Yet beyond the factors specific to how LHCPs will be designed, there are externalities that could make or break the success of the Dream Plan. Given the breadth of the Dream Plan, myriad regulatory, political, and social issues must be appreciated.

THE PRIVATE SECTOR MUST LEAD IMPLEMENTATION

The Dream Plan, particularly the LHCP, will require significant shifts in consumer behavior, societal thinking, health care delivery, and regulatory policies. It is impossible to predict whether these changes will take place in totality, whether other changes may be required, or the specific dates by which any of these shifts may come to fruition. The Dream Plan serves as a starting point, a blueprint for change that must be proposed, reworked, and value-tested so it can evolve into a practical, effective solution. Creativity, flexibility, diligence, and a long-term vision will be essential operational factors that will influence the success of the plan. That is why the transition of the Dream Plan from theory to reality must be spearheaded by the private sector, not by the government.

If we've learned anything from the failure of the Affordable Care Act, it is that the government should never legislate comprehensive, untested ideas intended to impact consumer behavior in the health care sector (and maybe in every other sector too, but that's a topic for a different book). Why? Because the government and economists cannot accurately predict how people will behave or what they will do.

Lawmakers rely on financial projections of proposed legislation to help them understand the potential impact these laws might have on taxes, the deficit, debt, and other major economic indicators. But when the laws don't work as expected, we're still stuck with the laws. We're stuck with the failed tax policies associated with the laws. On top of those burdens, we still haven't fixed the problem that the laws were intended to address.

The projections that the CBO makes on proposed legislation are akin to what one might see in the business plan of a start-up. Both analyses use historical information, expert advice, and projections of the future to determine potential outcomes. Rarely does a start-up execute exactly what's in the business plan—especially as the years go by. And it shouldn't. The company must react to the market, change course, and modify its plans. The government cannot behave this way because it is bound by the regulations established before anyone could know what would actually happen.

That's why the CBO's projections incorrectly estimated the value that the ACA would bring to the American people.[1] The law impacted so many aspects of both business and regulatory environments, and it made myriad assumptions about individual behavior that were essential to the program's success. When certain events did not manifest as expected, such as when some states did not expand Medicaid and when individuals accepted the financial penalties for violating the individual mandate, many of the program's underlying assumptions became invalid. Rates went up in many markets, not down. Millions of Americans remained uninsured.

Instead of overseeing large-scale transformative efforts, the government should serve as a cooperative partner to America's innovators and leaders. Broad-based acceptance of the LHCP will be enhanced if consumers feel confident that their data is being protected, their money is being managed professionally, and the program has been reviewed and accepted by the appropriate regulatory agents. At the same time, the government must afford LHCP developers the freedom to test market strategies and restructure certain legislation and rules to allow for the most effective rollout of the program.

REGULATORS MUST BE PROACTIVELY MANAGED

The LHCP is a disruptive, innovative product. It's never been implemented anywhere in the world. That means that all the protections identified above related to data security, medical safety, and money management have not be stipulated. Regulators will be anxious to monitor LHCPs and may be aggressive in passing legislation that could impact the effectiveness of the products.

For example, regulators could dictate data security requirements that could be overly costly to implement or could impede the product's capabilities. LHCP companies may have to provide compliance reports that are onerous to produce, given how data may be organized by the company. The feds could require minimum medical coverage requirements for certain diseases and conditions that would run contrary to the clinical protocols designed by some LHCP customers. All of these actions could restrict the speed and responsiveness that LHCP companies will need as they bring these new products to the market. Even more concerning, they could negatively impact the quality of LHCP outcomes.

Another key issue may relate to how an LHCP is classified. This, in turn, may affect the rules that govern it. For example, one could argue that the LHCP is an investment product. Were that to be the case, regulations associated with monitoring the financial services industry would apply to the LHCP. Alternatively, one could argue that the LHCP is a form of insurance. Such a judgment would put the LHCP under the purview of federal, state, and local insurance regulations. It could get complicated.

It is essential that LHCP developers acknowledge these issues during the early stages of product development. LHCPs could sustain a significant blow to their credibility if, after several years of robust adoption, regulatory agencies make the products subject to rules that could fundamentally alter their effectiveness and profitability. A proactive management of regulatory agents will be necessary to ensure that LHCP products can be both disruptive and legal.

INDIVIDUALS MUST BE FREE TO TRANSITION OUT OF PRIVATE INSURANCE AND MEDICARE

The LHCP will be a substitute for private insurance and Medicare. Odds are that the rollout of the LHCP will happen faster than any policy changes that might impact LHCP enrollees' ability to opt out of mandated health insurance programs or Medicare. As a result, in the early years of LHCP implementation, some LHCP enrollees may be "doubly insured."

Employers will likely be pressured to provide the individuals who are enrolled in an LHCP with a financial contribution commensurate to the employer-sponsored insurance benefits accessed by employees who do not have an LHCP. Many LHCP enrollees will need these funds as a key component of their LHCP savings. It is unclear how the role of the employer as health insurance subsidizer will play out as LHCPs evolve, but the issue is sure to be contentious.

Even more contentious will be the legal exemption of LHCP enrollees from the Medicare program. This may be one of the thorniest issues to tackle politically, legislatively, financially, and operationally. In the early years of LHCP rollout, individuals may still wind up paying payroll and other direct Medicare taxes even if they don't participate in the program. Yet at some point, if individuals will not be using Medicare services, they should be exempt from paying into the program.

That said, LHCP enrollees will still need to contribute to public health for the needy. Just how much they contribute today versus what will be needed to fund these programs tomorrow will require a massive audit of how tax dollars for Medicare and Medicaid are collected, invested, and spent. That could take years.

Even the Social Security payment process may need to change. Similar to the payroll tax, a Medicare tax is applied to Social Security payments. These funds should not be debited from the accounts of LHCP participants, as they would not be using Medicare services. Restructuring policy to allow for these and other changes will require a groundswell of consumer support for LHCP products. The more these products are adapted by Americans, the more public demand there will be to restructure the laws that support them.

MARKET-BASED PRICING MUST BE IDENTIFIED

The American health care system has a funky relationship with the word *cost*. It is used interchangeably with *price*, *reimbursement*, *payment*, and *expense,* depending on who's using it. Those who are paying out dollars for health care goods and services (the government and payers) tend to use the words cost and expense. When Medicare reduces the rates it pays to providers or reduces spending in a part of the program, CMS claims that it has "reduced costs." But from the provider's perspective, CMS has reduced the reimbursement or the payments it receives.

Over 80% of hospitals are not-for-profit or community entities, so they're not in the business, so to speak, of making money. Their perspective on their operations is a zero-sum game. As long as the reimbursement they receive covers their operational or variable costs, all is well. Traditionally, they use donations, grants, and other government payments (like DSH payments) to cover overhead, capital expenditures, and other so-called fixed costs.

This thinking has caused many providers to view the reimbursement that they receive as equivalent to the operational costs that are required to deliver the care. As a result, many hospitals don't really know the true cost of care in their facilities because they don't allocate their fixed costs to the different cases or procedures or drugs that they use. The issue is so systemic that one study revealed that about 90% of hospital CFOs do not have a handle on their organization's cost structure.[2]

This problem has been exacerbated by the fact that most providers do not use cost accounting systems. EMRs are clinical and billing systems. They require users to electronically check off all the necessary clinical activities that will enable the provider to get paid for the encounter, procedure, or test. Therefore, the best data that a provider can get on an encounter, procedure, or test is associated with the codes for each of these per-unit activities. And codes are associated with charge masters and reimbursement rate charts, not with costs.

All of this matters to an LHCP enrollee because he or she will be engaging directly with providers to pay for care. Providers will need to come up with prices they can charge that will cover their costs. If providers don't have a comprehensive understanding of how variable and fixed costs are allocated to the care they deliver, then they can't make an informed decision about how to price services.

As outlined in the Care Costing description of the LHCP in

chapter 8, direct-to-provider pricing has started to work its way into different segments of the industry, especially on the outpatient side. Activities are less complicated so they're easier to price. LHCP customers can already find market-based pricing for primary care visits, lab tests, and many outpatient surgical procedures.

It's going to take a Herculean effort for hospitals to embrace market-based pricing because of the variability in costs associated with the acute (more complicated) care they deliver. The cost for a kidney transplant for a healthy young man should be less than it would be for a diabetic older woman. Hospitals are going to have to use some health and demographic data, such as age, sex, and comorbidities (other conditions of the patient), to create a range of potential costs for major services in a market-based environment.

The challenge will come when the ultimate costs exceed the highest range quoted to a customer before the care was delivered. There may be completely legitimate, medical reasons why estimates may be inaccurate, such as unexpected surgical complications. On the flip side, padded and unnecessary services may have been added to the patient's bill. A hospital or industry-based review board will need to be developed to adjudicate these cases.

Identifying retail prices for pharmaceuticals will be a separate and equally challenging issue, as the drug industry is subject to its own norms and peccadillos. As discussed in chapter 9, the supply chain in the pharmaceutical industry makes web-like connections between drug manufacturers, wholesale distributors, group purchasing organizations, and virtually every hybrid buyer/manager/seller that could be imagined. There are volume discounts, rebate programs, and subsidy programs, all of which contribute to the difficulty in understanding what any of these drugs should actually cost.

As noted earlier, a likely solution would be for an LHCP member group to develop its own pharmacy benefits manager (PBM). It would be able to purchase drugs directly from manufacturers and provide them to participants.

As challenging as these issues may seem, they're not insurmountable. Shifting to cost-based pricing should benefit providers, because they will have much better management data that could be used to improve operations and lower costs. Simplifying the drug supply chain could reduce costs to LHCP members and provide a benchmark for other purchasers of drugs. This type of change should be embraced by every constituent in the industry, whether the Dream Plan is a success or not.

RATE CUTTING BY THE GOVERNMENT MUST BE PROHIBITED

If budgeted dollars become tight, then the administering agencies should limit the number of services provided to those enrolled in public health. Priority for care, assuming all else was equal, would be given to those who completed work or volunteer requirements and/or individuals who engaged in an annual well check with their primary care doctor.

What needs to be prohibited in this scenario is a strategy used by the government today to control costs: rate cutting.

In the Dream Plan, providers will be publishing competitive rates for services. These prices are those that individuals will be paying out of pocket for their care. If the government undercuts providers and pays them at lower rates, then LHCP enrollees will ostensibly subsidize public health at the transaction level. Providers will have to increase the rates they charge to retail (LHCP) customers to make up for the losses they sustain because of the government's lower rates.

This, by the way, is what happens today when commercial insurers reimburse providers at rates higher than the government. The phenomenon will just be much more transparent in a retail environment.

Further, government price cuts to providers might unjustifiably benefit those on public health. The Dream Plan supposes that the care plans of LHCP users will be used as the basis for plans for public health enrollees with similar health profiles. All the health needs of a certain type of LHCP user would be identified. The costs—the retail, market-based costs that an LHCP enrollee would pay—would be attached to these care needs. The sum of the costs for these services is the designated amount that government can spend on the care for an individual enrolled in public health.

If the government takes that sum and then demands rate cuts from providers, then the amount of care that's provided to those on public health could be greater than what individuals are paying for out of pocket on an LHCP. This unjustly penalizes Americans enrolled in an LHCP.

Some providers may simply refuse to take a rate cut from the government, as they do today. This is easier to do in the outpatient environment, where doctors and providers can sustain their businesses with payments only from private insurers. Hospitals don't have that luxury. Right now, much of the care delivered in hospitals today is to older, sicker Americans—most of whom are enrolled in Medicare. This makes hospitals financially dependent on Medicare for survival, even when CMS cuts its rates.

But the Dream Plan would allow Americans to opt out of Medicare and pay hospitals directly for care at rates established by the facility. The payment process for the hospital would be significantly simplified, reducing costs and potentially improving their financial position. Some hospitals may reach a tipping point where they would be able to operate serving LHCP patients alone, and simply reject patients on government-funded programs if the government demands lower rates for care. The hospital system might then evolve into a two-tier system, with some accepting government-funded patients, and others accepting only LHCP patients.

One would expect that the hospital that charges more (meaning the one accepting LHCP patients) would have more resources to spend on infrastructure, on hiring the best doctors and staff, and on attracting the best management teams. Such advantages would almost certainly lead to higher outcomes for these patients. This should serve as a cautionary tale for government officials who want to ensure that individuals on public health are afforded the same access to high-quality care as everyone else. *Don't cut rates to providers.*

WE ALL NEED TO ADJUST OUR ATTITUDE

American Dreamers are self-sufficient, motivated, and goal-oriented. We are empowered to find ways to make positive change for ourselves and our families. In order for the Dream Plan to be successful across all sectors of society, our entire population must apply the American Dream philosophies to the management of our personal health. It is imperative that we change our view on what we consider healthy behavior, because we simply cannot afford the health care that we require today. Shifting our mindset about personal health is going to take some major cultural and sociological changes.

The Dream Plan seeks to incent individuals to improve their health by aligning our behaviors with our health care costs. The healthier we are, the lower our health care costs will be. Yet reducing costs cannot be the single motivator to improving the health of Americans. Wealthy individuals, who are not sensitive to the cost of care, may not make behavior changes to save money. Those on public health, whose care is subsidized by their fellow Americans, don't have a financial incentive to improve their health status either. And even those who are price sensitive may be influenced by other factors that can impact their health.

Our continued exposure to any activity, good or bad, makes the behavior seem normal. Improving our health will require us to break the cycles that cause us to adapt the negative and sometimes self-destructive behaviors of those around us. For example, we may be told that we are making poor choices when we overeat and stress out and rely on pain medications to get us through the day. But when those around us are engaging in similar activities, our motivation to break the cycle is weakened. Why be a social outcast for eating yogurt when you can enjoy ice cream like everyone around you?

Overworking is another badge of honor that's got to get its wings clipped. Worker productivity in America is at historic lows[3] and no one's quite sure why. Americans must learn to work more effectively, not just work more, because, evidently, working more doesn't mean we're actually getting more done. But it does mean we're adding to our own stress and depriving ourselves of sleep. Both of these issues are major contributors to poor health and must be addressed if we want our overall health status to improve.

The need to be healthy must become a definitive feature of being American. We need better role models in the media, and we need better messaging from social services. Corporate America should recognize that their bottom lines are impacted when their workers are stressed and less productive. We need to motivate ourselves and encourage each other to improve because healthy Americans will lead happier, healthier, and more productive lives.

CHAPTER 14

RECOMMENDATIONS FOR SHORT-TERM CHANGE

The timeline will be long before the Dream Plan comes to complete fruition, yet the American health care system needs change right now. There are a lot of ideas that could be implemented today that would lay the foundation for a successful Dream Plan tomorrow.

The ideas outlined below would largely affect policy. Changes to current laws would be necessary to bring these proposals to bear. Given Congress's struggle to work cooperatively on almost any issue, achieving some of these ideas may seem unattainable. Nonetheless, there are strong leaders and supporters of health care reform both in and outside of government who should be debating new ideas and continuing their efforts to lobby for change.

MANDATE ANNUAL PRIMARY CARE VISITS FOR ALL AMERICANS

The effective use of primary care is an essential part of a well-functioning health care system. As discussed at length in this book, patients and primary care providers must collaborate closely to develop customized health plans. Patients will be more engaged in their health if they know their doctor is prescribing the treatments that are tailored for their needs.

In addition, regular visits to a PCP ensure that an individual's health record is updated with recent information. Doctors can spot trends and identify potential issues before they escalate if they are provided with a robust set of patient information. Visits to a primary care doctor don't only help the individual patient, they also help the community. Public health officials can do a better job of managing public health if primary care data is available from everyone.

MANDATE WORKER REQUIREMENTS FOR MEDICAID ENROLLEES

Work and volunteer requirements for Medicaid enrollees is becoming increasingly popular in states across the country. States that previously resisted the Medicaid expansion authorized by the ACA, like Virginia, have been able to win over supporters by attaching these requirements to their Medicaid programs.

As noted earlier, a significant number of Medicaid enrollees already work, so the requirement should not be onerous to the majority of beneficiaries. Yet it does emphasize the responsibility that each of us has in contributing to the greater good. Mandating that individuals work, volunteer, or look for opportunities to do either benefits all Americans.

RATION CARE IN PUBLIC
HEALTH PROGRAMS

The budgets for Medicare and Medicaid have been expanding at alarming rates, and the financial mandate for change in these programs has been made clear. Using rate-cutting tactics can only pull so many costs out of the system. We also have to cut back on the number of services being provided. That means care has to be rationed more effectively.

All the arguments used to support rationing in the Dream Plan can be applied to our Medicaid and Medicare programs. Basic services that all enrollees would be entitled to receive must be defined, much like they are today. Costs for expensive care and drugs should be tracked and compared against budgeted spending to make sure cost overruns don't occur. More than likely, toward the end of a period, certain services will have to be put off for selected individuals.

The system should also use the annual primary care visit and worker requirements as a means to ration care. This may be more applicable to Medicaid enrollees than to those on Medicare. Many Medicare enrollees cannot work due to their age and health condition. And many of them see their primary care doctor on a regular basis as it is.

That makes rationing in the Medicare environment much more challenging. One of the key roadblocks relates to the fact that older people, who are on Medicare, are more likely to vote. And they're not going to like rationed services.

Family members and loved ones can help lower costs by proactively managing the health care needs of the elderly as they approach the end of their lives. This is especially relevant for those who lose their cognitive capabilities. All Americans should be encouraged to talk about how they want to die before death is imminent so they can make important decisions as objectively as possible. In addition, the medical and regulatory communities must do a better job of incorporating patient and family preferences in treatment options.

Perhaps one of the best ways to ease into rationing Medicare services is to reduce the size of the program by allowing individuals to opt out. Odds are that the folks who would initially opt out of Medicare would be healthier and wealthier than the average enrollee. As more people opt out of the program, the remaining pool is likely to be less wealthy and less healthy than it was initially. But it will be smaller, and hopefully, easier to manage.

One would hope that shrinking the size of the Medicare program should help make the rationing process more fair. Right now, a physician's opinion related to a patient's medical need is a key driver that determines whether the patient can access certain drugs, surgeries, etc. Advancements in research and technology have brought an incredible array of new drugs and therapies to the market. We've reached a point where medical necessity is becoming an invalid rationale to approve access to care because such an approach creates a financially untenable program.

Some approaches to rationing, such as using age as a criterion, developing a lottery system, or approving therapies for patients whose health profile demonstrates the best odds of success, will need to be incorporated into the Medicare system. With fewer patients to cover (assuming some are able to opt out), CMS has an opportunity to develop rationing criteria for a more manageable group of enrollees. The issue of fairly controlling access to the explosion of care options for Medicare enrollees is probably the most critical concern that CMS will have to address in the coming years.

REQUIRE UNIVERSAL HEALTH INSURANCE COVERAGE

Despite the efforts of the ACA, about 16% of adult non-elderly Americans still have no health insurance. With the repeal of the individual mandate in 2017, the number of uninsured is expected to increase. This is a worrisome trend, because all Americans should have health insurance coverage. Those who do not buy insurance and wind up incurring significant health care expenses can put themselves in financial peril. Having health insurance makes sure that no one is at risk of financial ruin as a result of a catastrophic medical event.

In addition, those who opt out of the insurance market and

generate high health care expenses can negatively impact their fellow citizens who have to pick up the tab. That burdens the entire health care ecosystem. Put simply, it's irresponsible for Americans not to have health insurance.

ELIMINATE THE TEN ESSENTIAL BENEFITS MANDATED BY ACA

As I've noted throughout this book, the ten essential benefits requirement of the ACA has inflated the cost of health insurance because enrollees are forced to pay for health coverage options they do not need or want. Many argue that eliminating this requirement will divide the marketplace into healthy and nonhealthy individuals, requiring sicker Americans to pay more for their care. Those who are healthy will not need many benefits, and they'll opt for plans with less coverage, which should, in turn, be cheaper. This would certainly be the case if the market stayed as small as it is today. But what if we could make it bigger?

ELIMINATE EMPLOYER-SPONSORED HEALTH INSURANCE

Americans have come to expect that a perk of full-time employment is access to an employer-sponsored health insurance plan. As noted previously, the federal government loses approximately $260 billion a year because employer-sponsored health insurance benefits are not taxed. Yet this isn't the main reason that the program should be eliminated (or at least modified).

The ACA market is in shambles because healthy individuals can opt out of buying care, the ten essential benefits requirement makes insurance more expensive than it has to be, and critically, many people in the market are sicker and less wealthy than those in employer-sponsored programs. If employer-sponsored health insurance were eliminated, the ACA market would increase by over ten times its current size. An influx of this magnitude into the ACA marketplace could provide enough healthy and wealthy buyers to subsidize the care for the lower income and/or less healthy individuals buying insurance.

This approach doesn't mean that employers will stop subsidizing the cost of health care for their employees. Rather, the intent is that employers will provide their employees with the resources they'll need to buy health care insurance on the open market instead of providing the health care insurance through their respective organizations.

This plan would be especially effective if the individual mandate is reinstated, requiring everyone to buy insurance. In addition, the ten essential benefits requirement should be lifted. Doing so would allow a wider variety of plans to be offered in this newly expanded market, offering something for everyone.

ALLOW MEDICARE TO NEGOTIATE WITH BIG PHARMA

A friendly reminder: current law stipulates that the Department of Health and Human Services cannot negotiate directly with drug companies on behalf of Medicare beneficiaries.

Interestingly, other government programs, including Medicaid and the Veterans Administration, are permitted to negotiate prices. Efforts to have Medicare take such a stance have had limited success because many argue that any reductions in pricing for one group of buyers will result in an increase in pricing for another. If the prices that Medicare pays go down, then potentially the price for consumers in other sectors will go up. While that makes sense in theory, it's hard to know which drugs would be impacted, which consumer buyers would be affected, and what the magnitude of the price increase would be.

The main reason that Medicare should be permitted to negotiate with Big Pharma is to eliminate price fixing. No aspect of the health care industry should be impacted by price fixing because it inhibits the functioning of a free market economy. We will never understand what the true market-derived price of drugs will be if prices for a significant portion of the spending is controlled by the manufacturers. It's time to change this legislation so we can push for more clarity on drug prices in America.

IMPROVE OUT-OF-NETWORK CHARGES FOR CASH-PAYING CUSTOMERS

One of the biggest challenges in implementing the Dream Plan is the requirement that hospitals provide direct-to-consumer pricing. Right now, when an individual has to pay cash, they are often charged rates from the charge master which, as discussed, are inflated. Patients have no idea what the right pricing should be. And neither do hospitals. But we can all agree that any prices from a charge master are wrong.

Individuals who do not have access to insurance, are satisfying deductibles, or opt to pay cash for services should not be penalized by providers by paying a higher rate than others for care. These individuals should have access at least to the average rate negotiated by the provider for contracted services with private insurers. Cash-paying customers warrant these lower-than-price-list rates because the payment processing for cash payments is much lower than it is for other insured customers.

As the health care industry shifts more and more to consumer-driven services, providers must remember that cash is king. Establishing policies that ensure fair charges for cash-paying customers makes the health care payment process much more equitable.

CONCLUSION

Americans are clamoring for a health care system that treats them with fairness and dignity. The Dream Plan offers Americans many of the things that they want, just packaged in a completely novel way.

Unlike our current health care system, the Dream Plan has been developed to evolve over time. It acknowledges that as individuals, we change over time. The plan takes into account the continuous flow of economic, personal, and physiological milestones that impact our lives. It is a flexible, disciplined system that mandates the longitudinal engagement in our health care experience.

The Dream Plan sets up the American health care system to be the most democratic in the world. Imagine a time when the vast majority of Americans have been enrolled in a Longitudinal Health Care Plan. Collectively, the data contained in these plans would represent the care preferences of the American populace. The information would demonstrate the choices Americans make when faced with end-of-life decisions. It would identify what trade-offs we're willing to make when resources are constrained. And critically, it would document how preventive care could improve the health and financial status of our citizenry.

This information could be used by the government as a model for how the public health system would be structured. In that way, the most democratic principles would be used in the creation of a public health program. The truly needy would have the opportunity to access the care that the average American had designed for him or herself.

Further, benchmarking programs could be in place that would allow similar individuals from all over America to compare plans. Americans could even compete with each other to lower their costs or to improve their outcomes. If that would happen, the Dream Plan wouldn't only disrupt the health care, insurance, and financial services industries, it would also impact gaming. Imagine an app where diabetic patients of similar demographic profiles compete to improve health outcomes by dietary modifications, weight loss, exercise regimes . . . The power of technology could be used to spur positive patient behavior in ways we've never seen before.

And let's not forget the rest of the world. The Dream Plan may be the first American health care delivery model that could be adapted by other countries. Because the Dream Plan is independent of the American payment system, it could become a universal standard for personal health care management. There's every possibility for the LHCP to be deployed anywhere from Dublin to Dubai. After we prove the technologies in America, we can take them around the globe.

World: Meet the American health care system.

NOTES

INTRODUCTION: THE ER: A CASE STUDY IN MISALIGNED INCENTIVES

1. "Emergency Medical Treatment & Labor Act (EMTALA)," Centers for Medicare and Medicaid Services, accessed June 19, 2018, https://www.cms.gov/regulations-and-guidance/legislation/emtala/index.html.

2. "First Look at Health Insurance Coverage in 2018 Finds ACA Gains Beginning to Reverse," Sara R. Collins, Munira Z. Gunja, Michelle M. Doty, and Herman K. Bhupal, The Commonwealth Fund, May 1, 2018, http://www.common wealthfund.org/publications/blog/2018/apr/health-coverage-erosion.

3. "The Burden of Medical Debt: Results from the Kaiser Family Foundation/New York Times Medical Bills Survey," Liz Hamel et al., Kaiser Family Foundation, January 5, 2016, https://www.kff.org/health-costs/report/the-burden-of-medical-debt-results-from-the-kaiser-family-foundationnew-york-times-medical-bills-survey/view/print.

4. "State Balance Billing Legislation Update," American College of Radiology, March 21, 2018, https://www.acr.org/advocacy-and-economics/advocacy-news/advocacy-news-issues/in-the-march-24-2018-issue/state-balance-billing-legislation-update.

5. "Direct-to-Consumer Telehealth May Increase Access to Care but Does Not Decrease Spending," J. Scott Ashwood et al., Rand Corporation, March 28, 2017, https://www.rand.org/pubs/external_publications/EP67074.html.

6. "In 3 States, If Anthem Thinks You Shouldn't Have Gone To ER, It Won't Pay," Robert Glatter, *Forbes*, October 16, 2017, https://www.forbes.com/sites/robertglatter/2017/10/16/anthem-at-odds-with-your-decision-to-visit-the-er-and-refusing-to-pay-in-certain-states/#5c02a9594356.

7. "Alternatives for 'Potentially Preventable' NYS Hospital ER Visits Examined," Blue Cross Blue Shield, April 6, 2016, https://www.bcbs.com/news/press-releases/alternatives-potentially-preventable-nys-hospital-er-visits-examined.

8. "Urgent Care Needs Among Nonurgent Visits to the Emergency Department," Renee Y. Hsia, MD, MSc; Ari B. Friedman, MS; Matthew Niedzwiecki, PhD, *JAMA*, June 2016, https://jamanetwork.com/journals/jamainternalmedicine/fullarticle/2515063.

9. "CMS Has Higher Penalties for Readmissions Than for Deaths," Tim Casey, *Cardiovascular Business*, October 26, 2016, https://www.cardiovascularbusiness.com/topics/healthcare-economics-policy/cms-has-higher-penalties-readmissions-deaths.

CHAPTER 1: HEALTH CARE PRIMER: UNDERSTANDING HEALTH CARE'S UNIQUE LANGUAGE

1. "Status of the ACA Medicaid Expansion after Supreme Court Ruling," Center on Budget and Policy Priorities, accessed June 30, 2018, https://www.cbpp.org/sites/default/files/atoms/files/status-of-the-ACA-medicaid-expansion-after-supreme-court-ruling.pdf.

2. "National Federation of Independent Business et al. v. Sebelius," Supreme Court of the United States, October 2011, https://www.supremecourt.gov/opinions/11pdf/11-393c3a2.pdf.

3. "Status of State Action on the Medicaid Expansion Decision," Kaiser Family Foundation, June 7, 2018, https://www.kff.org/health-reform/state-indicator/state-activity-around-expanding-medicaid-under-the-affordable-care-act/.

4. "2018 Obamacare Subsidy Calculator," Healthinsurance.org, June 29, 2018, https://www.healthinsurance.org/obamacare/subsidy-calculator/.

5. "Uninsured with Traumatic Injuries May Be Cured into Destitution," Ronnie Cohen, Reuters, April 20, 2017, https://www.reuters.com/article/us-health-injury-bankruptcy-idUSKBN17M2SB.

6. "Mike Pence Says Under Obamacare, 'American Families Have Seen an Increase in Premiums of $5,000,'" Louis Jacobson, Politifact, January 9, 2017, http://www.politifact.com/truth-o-meter/statements/2017/jan/09/mike-pence/mike-pence-says-under-obamacare-american-families-/.

7. "Average Annual Workplace Family Health Premiums Rise Modest 3% to $18,142 in 2016; More Workers Enroll in High-Deductible Plans With Savings Option Over Past Two Years," Kaiser Family Foundation, September 14, 2016, https://www.kff.org/health-costs/press-release/average-annual-workplace-family-health-premiums-rise-modest-3-to-18142-in-2016-more-workers-enroll-in-high-deductible-plans-with-savings-option-over-past-two-years/.

8. "Health Savings Accounts and High Deductible Health Plans Grow as Valuable Financial Planning Tools," America's Health Insurance Plans, April 2018, https://www.ahip.org/wp-content/uploads/2018/04/HSA_Report_4.12.18.pdf.

9. "What Medicare Covers," Medicare.gov, accessed June 19, 2018, https://www.medicare.gov/what-medicare-covers/index.html.

10. "The Facts on Medicare Spending and Financing," Juliette Cubanski and Tricia Neuman, Kaiser Family Foundation, June 22, 2018, https://www.kff.org/medicare/issue-brief/the-facts-on-medicare-spending-and-financing/.

11. "An Aging Nation: The Older Population in the United States," Jennifer M. Ortman, Victoria A. Velkoff, and Howard Hogan, U.S. Census Bureau, issued May 2014, https://www.census.gov/prod/2014pubs/p25-1140.pdf.

12. "Medicare Financial Outlook Worsens," Phil Galewitz, Kaiser Health News, June 5, 2018, https://khn.org/news/medicare-financial-outlook-worsens/.

13. "How Do Medicare Advantage Plans Work?" Medicare.gov, accessed June 19, 2018, https://www.medicare.gov/sign-up-change-plans/medicare-health-plans/medicare-advantage-plans/how-medicare-advantage-plans-work.html.

14. "What's Medicare Supplement Insurance (Medigap)?" Medicare.gov, accessed June 19, 2018, https://www.medicare.gov/supplement-other-insurance/medigap/whats-medigap.html.

15. "Distribution of Lifetime Medicare Taxes and Spending by Sex and by Lifetime Household Earnings," Xiaotong Niu, Congressional Budget Office, August 2017, https://www.cbo.gov/system/files/115th-congress-2017-2018/workingpaper/52985-workingpaper.pdf.

16. "Policy Basics: Introduction to Medicaid," Center on Budget and Policy Priorities, last updated August 16, 2016, http://www.cbpp.org/research/health/policy-basics-introduction-to-medicaid.

17. "Medicaid Cuts May Force Retirees Out of Nursing Homes," Jordan Rau, *The New York Times*, June 24, 2017, https://www.nytimes.com/2017/06/24/science/medicaid-cutbacks-elderly-nursing-homes.html.

18. "Medicaid and CHIP: Strengthening Coverage, Improving Health," Centers for Medicare and Medicaid Services, January 2017, https://www.medicaid.gov/medicaid/program-information/downloads/accomplishments-report.pdf.

19. "Underpayment by Medicare and Medicaid Fact Sheet, December 2017 Update," American Hospital Association, accessed June 30, 2018, https://www.aha.org/statistics/2018-01-03-underpayment-medicare-and-medicaid-fact-sheet-december-2017-update.

20. "Summary of Research: Medicaid Physician Payment and Access to Care," American Medical Association, accessed June 19, 2018, https://www.ama-assn.org/sites/default/files/media-browser/public/arc/research-summary-medicaid-physician-payment_0.pdf.

21. "Significant Primary Care, Overall Physician Shortage Predicted by 2025," American Academy of Family Physicians, March 23, 2015, https://www.aafp.org/news/practice-professional-issues/2015 0303aamcwkforce.html.

22. "Top 10 Causes of Deaths in India," *The Times of India*, September 20, 2017, https://timesofindia.indiatimes.com/india/what-are-the-top-10-causes-of-death-in-india/articleshow/60762113.cms.

23. "Air Pollution More Deadly in Africa Than Malnutrition or Dirty Water, Study Warns," *The Guardian*, accessed June 30, 2018, https://www.theguardian.com/global-development/2016/oct/20/air-pollution-deadlier-africa-than-dirty-water-or-malnutrition-oecd.

CHAPTER 2: THE MONEY: WHERE IT ALL GOES

1. "NHE Fact Sheet," Centers for Medicare and Medicaid Services, last modified April 17, 2018, https://www.cms.gov/research-statistics-data-and-systems/statistics-trends-and-reports/nationalhealthexpenddata/nhe-fact-sheet.html. This figure is compiled by the Centers for Medicare and Medicaid Services, CMS, in conjunction with various data gathering organizations.

2. "National Health Expenditure Accounts: Methodology Paper, 2016 Definitions, Sources, and Methods," Centers for Medicare and Medicaid Services, accessed July 1, 2018, https://www.cms.gov/research-statistics-data-and-systems/statistics-trends-and-reports/nationalhealthexpenddata/downloads/dsm-16.pdf.

3. Other Programs includes worksite health care, other private revenues, Indian Health Service, workers' compensation, general assistance, maternal and child health, vocational rehabilitation, other federal programs, Substance Abuse and Mental Health Services Administration, other state and local programs, and school health. Other Insurance includes CHIP, Department of Defense, and Department of Veterans Affairs.

4. Premiums paid out of pocket for insurance are included in the Private Insurance or Medicare categories, depending on the enrollee.

5. From the Kaiser Family Foundation. https://www.kff.org.

6. In other sections of this book, I quote the uninsured rate at almost 16%. That figure is for the first quarter of 2018 and refers to the percentage of adult non-elderly Americans. The 9% uninsured rate shown here is for all Americans for 2016. Other Public includes those covered in the military and under the Veterans Administration.

7. "Report for Selected Countries and Subjects," International Monetary Fund, accessed July 5, 2018, http://www.imf.org/external/pubs/ft/weo/2018/01/weodata/weorept.aspx?pr.x=69&pr.y=15&sy=2016&ey=2018&scsm=1&ssd=1&sort=country&ds=.&br=1&c=134&s=NGDP%2CNGDPD&grp=0&a=.

8. "The Federal Budget in 2016," Congressional Budget Office, accessed July 1, 2018, https://www.cbo.gov/sites/default/files/115th-congress-2017-2018/graphic/52408-budget overall.pdf. Discretionary Spending (Non-Defense) includes spending on certain programs related to transportation, education, veterans' benefits, health, housing assistance, and other activities. Other includes spending on unemployment compensation, federal civilian and military retirement, some veterans' benefits, the earned income tax credit, the Supplemental Nutrition Assistance Program, and other mandatory programs, minus income from offsetting receipts.

9. "The 2017 Long-Term Budget Outlook," Congressional Budget Office, March 30, 2017, https://www.cbo.gov/publication/52480.

10. "The World Factbook," Central Intelligence Agency, accessed July 1, 2018, https://www.cia.gov/library/publications/the-world-factbook/fields/2222.html.

11. "Mortality in the United States, 2015," Jiaquan Xu, MD, Sherry L. Murphy, BS, Kenneth D. Kochanek, MA, and Elizabeth Arias, PhD, U.S. Department of Health and Human Services, December 2016, https://www.cdc.gov/nchs/data/databriefs/db267.pdf.

12. "Mortality in the United States, 2016," Kenneth D. Kochanek, MA, Sherry L. Murphy, BS, Jiaquan Xu, MD, and Elizabeth Arias, PhD., U.S. Department of

Health and Human Services, December 2017, https://www.cdc.gov/nchs/data/databriefs/db293.pdf. The life expectancy for 2015 was listed as 78.8 years in the December 2016 NCHS Data Brief. The figure for 2015 life expectancy was revised to 78.7 in the December 2017 NCHS Data Brief.

13. "Life Expectancy and Healthy Life Expectancy Data by Country," World Health Organization, last updated April 6, 2018, http://apps.who.int/gho/data/node.main.688. Note that the life expectancy for the United States in Chart 6 is 78.5 years. The source of the data in the chart is the World Health Organization. Their calculation of life expectancy differs from the source cited earlier, which pegs life expectancy in America for 2016 at 78.6.

14. "Why U.S. Women Still Die During Childbirth," Alexandra Sifferlin, *Time*, September 27, 2016, http://time.com/4508369/why-u-s-women-still-die-during-childbirth/.

15. "U.S. Has the Worst Rate of Maternal Deaths in the Developed World," Nina Martin and Renee Montagne, NPR, May 12, 2017, https://www.npr.org/2017/05/12/528098789/u-s-has-the-worst-rate-of-maternal-deaths-in-the-developed-world.

16. "'We Should Be Really Alarmed': U.S. Life Expectancy Drops Due to Staggering Rate of Overdose Deaths," Kaiser Health News, December 21, 2017, https://khn.org/morning-breakout/we-should-be-really-alarmed-u-s-life-expectancy-drops-due-to-staggering-rate-of-overdose-deaths/.

17. "Overdose Deaths Involving Opioids, Cocaine, and Psychostimulants—United States, 2015–2016," Puja Seth et al., Centers for Disease Control, March 30, 2018, https://www.cdc.gov/mmwr/volumes/67/wr/mm6712a1.htm?s_cid=mm6712a1_w.

18. "Drug Overdose Death Data," Centers for Disease Control, accessed June 19, 2018, https://www.cdc.gov/drugoverdose/data/statedeaths.html.

19. "U.S. Maker of Oxycontin Painkiller to Pay $600 Million in Guilty Plea," Barry Meier, *The New York Times*, May 11, 2007, https://www.nytimes.com/2007/05/11/business/worldbusiness/11iht-oxy.1.5665287.html.

20. "Adult Obesity Facts," Centers for Disease Control, accessed June 19, 2018, https://www.cdc.gov/obesity/data/adult.html.

21. E.A. Finkelstein, J.G. Trogdon, J.W. Cohen, and W. Dietz, "Annual Medical Spending Attributable to Obesity: Payer-and Service-Specific Estimates," *Health Affairs* 28, no. 5 (2009): w822–831.

22. "Health, United States, 2016 - Individual Charts and Tables: Spreadsheet, PDF, and PowerPoint Files," Table 058, accessed July 2, 2018, https://www.cdc.gov/nchs/hus/contents2016.htm#healthriskfactors, Centers for Disease Control.

23. "Fewer Americans in This Decade Want to Lose Weight," Art Swift, Gallup, November 22, 2016, https://news.gallup.com/poll/198074/fewer-americans -lose-weight-past-decade.aspx.

24. "Obesity Update," Organisation for Economic Co-operation and Development, accessed July 1, 2018, https://www.oecd.org/els/health-systems/Obesity-Update-2017.pdf.

25. "Childhood Obesity Facts," Centers for Disease Control, accessed June 19, 2018, https://www.cdc.gov/healthyschools/obesity/facts.htm.

CHAPTER 3: A HISTORICAL VIEW OF HEALTH POLICY: HOW DID THINGS GET SO COMPLICATED?

1. *Manly Health and Training: To Teach the Science of a Sound and Beautiful Body*, Walt Whitman, (New York: Regan Arts, 2017).

2. "A Brief History of the Antibiotic Era: Lessons Learned and Challenges for the Future," Rustam I. Aminov, *Frontiers in Microbiology* 1, (October 29, 2010): 134, https://www.ncbi.nlm.nih.gov/pmc/articles/PMC3109405/.

3. "Health Insurance in the United States," Melissa Thomasson, EH.net, accessed July 1, 2018, https://eh.net/encyclopedia/health-insurance-in-the-united-states/.

4. "History of Health Reform Efforts in the United States," Kaiser Family Foundation, March 25, 2011, https://www.kff.org/health-reform/timeline/ history-of-health-reform-efforts-in-the-united-states/.

5. "Key Elements of the U.S. Tax System," Tax Policy Center, accessed June 20, 2018, http://www.taxpolicycenter.org/briefing-book/how-does-tax-exclusion -employer-sponsored-health-insurance-work.

6. "A Look at the 1940 Census," U.S. Census Bureau, accessed July 1, 2018, https:// www.census.gov/newsroom/cspan/1940census/CSPAN_1940slides.pdf.

7. "Prevalence of Overweight, Obesity, and Extreme Obesity Among Adults: United States, Trends 1960–1962 Through 2007–2008," Centers for Disease Control, June 2010, https://www.cdc.gov/nchs/data/hestat/obesity_ adult_07_08/obesity_adult_07_08.pdf.

8. "A Milestone En Route to a Majority Minority Nation," Paul Taylor and D'Vera Cohn, Pew Research Center, November 7, 2012, http://www.pewsocialtrends. org/2012/11/07/a-milestone-en-route-to-a-majority-minority-nation/.

9. "Religious Diversity in America, 1940–2000," Michael Hout and Claude S. Fischer, Survey Research Center, University of California at Berkeley, August 2001, http://ucdata.berkeley.edu/rsfcensus/papers/Hout_FischerASA.pdf.

10. "NHE Fact Sheet," Centers for Medicare and Medicaid Services, accessed June

19, 2018, https://www.cms.gov/research-statistics-data-and-systems/statistics-trends-and-reports/nationalhealthexpenddata/nhe-fact-sheet.html.

11. "Clinton's Health Plan: The Overview," Robert Pear, *The New York Times*, accessed June 20, 2018, https://www.nytimes.com/1993/10/28/us/clinton-s-health-plan-overview-congress-given-clinton-proposal-for-health-care.html.

12. "Searching for Savings in Medicare Drug Price Negotiations," Juliette Cubanski and Tricia Neuman, Kaiser Family Foundation, April 26, 2018, https://www.kff.org/medicare/issue-brief/searching-for-savings-in-medicare-drug-price-negotiations/.

13. "Table 22. Life Expectancy at Birth, at Age 65, and at Age 75, by Sex, Race, and Hispanic Origin: United States, Selected Years 1900-2010," Centers for Disease Control, accessed July 1, 2018, https://www.cdc.gov/nchs/data/hus/2011/022.pdf.

CHAPTER 4: PERSPECTIVES ON HEALTH INSURANCE

1. "National Ambulatory Medical Care Survey: 2015 State and National Summary Tables," Centers for Disease Control, table 12, accessed July 1, 2018, https://www.cdc.gov/nchs/data/ahcd/namcs_summary/2015_namcs_web_tables.pdf.

2. "The Truth About the Uninsured Rate in America," Tami Luhby, CNN Money, March 14, 2017, http://money.cnn.com/2017/03/13/news/economy/uninsured-rate-obamacare/index.html.

3. "Improvements in Health Status after Massachusetts Health Care Reform," Philip J . Van der Wees, and Alan M. Zaslavsky, John Z. Ayanian, *Milbank Quarterly*, December 2013, https://www.milbank.org/quarterly/articles/improvements-in-health-status-after-massachusetts-health-care-reform/.

4. "Three-Year Impacts of the Affordable Care Act: Improved Medical Care and Health Among Low Income Adults," Benjamin D. Sommers et al., *Health Affairs*, June 2017, https://www.healthaffairs.org/doi/abs/10.1377/hlthaff.2017.0293.

5. "The Oregon Health Insurance Experiment," Katherine Baicker, PhD, et al., accessed June 20, 2018, http://www.nber.org/oregon/.

6. "Medicaid Expansion Wishes Aren't Coming True," Joel Zinberg, *U.S. News & World Report*, Oct. 26, 2016, https://www.usnews.com/opinion/policy-dose/articles/2016-10-26/oregons-medicaid-expansion-is-a-cautionary-tale-for-obamacare.

7. "Sounding Board: Health Insurance Coverage and Health—What the Recent

Evidence Tells Us," Benjamin D. Sommers, MD, PhD, Atul A. Gawande, MD, MPH, and Katherine Baicker, PhD, *New England Journal of Medicine* 377 (August 10, 2017), 586–593, https://www.nejm.org/doi/full/10.1056/nejmsb1706645.

8. "10 Leading Causes of Death by Age Group, United States – 2010," Centers for Disease Control, accessed July 1, 2018, https://www.cdc.gov/injury/wisqars/pdf/10lcid_all_deaths_by_age_group_2010-a.pdf.

9. "Inequalities in Life Expectancy Among US Counties, 1980 to 2014," Laura Dwyer Lindgren, MPH et al., *JAMA Internal Medicine* 177, no. 7 (July 2017): 1003–1011, https://jamanetwork.com/journals/jamainternalmedicine/article-abstract/2626194.

10. "Beyond Health Care: The Role of Social Determinants in Promoting Health and Health Equity," Samantha Artiga and Elizabeth Hinton, Kaiser Family Foundation, May 10, 2018, http://www.kff.org/disparities-policy/issue-brief/beyond-health-care-the-role-of-social-determinants-in-promoting-health-and-health-equity/.

11. "The Relative Contribution of Multiple Determinants to Health," *Health Affairs*, August 21, 2014, http://healthaffairs.org/healthpolicybriefs/brief_pdfs/healthpolicybrief_123.pdf.

12. "Social Determinants of Health: Know What Affects Health," Centers for Disease Control, accessed June 20, 2018, https://www.cdc.gov/socialdeterminants/.

13. "Dietary Salt Intake and Hypertension," Sung Kyu Ha, MD, *Electrolytes and Blood Pressure* 12, no. 1 (June 2014), 7–18, https://www.ncbi.nlm.nih.gov/pmc/articles/PMC4105387/.

14. "Ultra-Processed Food Linked to Cancer, Study Says," Jamie Ducharme, *Time*, Feb. 14, 2018, http://time.com/5157885/processed-foods-cancer/.

15. "Crohn's Disease," Mayo Clinic, accessed June 20, 2018, https://www.mayoclinic.org/diseases-conditions/crohns-disease/diagnosis-treatment/drc-20353309.

16. "Biologics," CCFA Facts Sheet, accessed June 20, 2018, http://www.crohnscolitisfoundation.org/assets/biologic-therapy.pdf.

CHAPTER 5: ATTEMPTS AT HEALTH
CARE TRANSFORMATION

1. "Savings in Electronic Medical Record Systems? Do It for the Quality," Clifford

Goodman, *Health Affairs* 24, no. 5 (September/October 2005), https://www.
healthaffairs.org/doi/full/10.1377/hlthaff.24.5.1124.

2. "CMS Has Taken Steps to Address Problems, but Needs to Further Implement
Systems Development Best Practices," U.S. Government Accountability Office,
March 2015, https://www.gao.gov/assets/670/668834.pdf.

3. "Tethered to the EHR: Primary Care Physician Workload Assessment Using
EHR Event Log Data and Time-Motion Observations," Brian G. Arndt, MD et
al., *Annals of Family Medicine* 15, no. 5 (September/October 2017): 419–426,
http://www.annfammed.org/content/15/5/419.full.

4. "Reviewing a Year of Serious Data Breaches, Major Attacks and New
Vulnerabilities," IBM Data Security, accessed July 1, 2018, https://www.
autoindustrylawblog.com/wp-content/uploads/sites/8/2016/05/IBM_2016-
cyber-security-intelligence-index.pdf.

5. "Doctors put patients in charge with Apple's Health Records feature," Apple.
com, March 29, 2018, https://www.apple.com/newsroom/2018/03/
doctors-put-patients-in-charge-with-apples-health-records-feature/.

CHAPTER 6: THE CASE AGAINST A SINGLE PAYER SYSTEM

1. "In U.S., Support for Government-Run Health System Edges Up," Frank
Newport, Gallup, December 1, 2017, https://news.gallup.com/poll/223031/
americans-support-government-run-health-system-edges.aspx.

2. "How Does Health Spending in the U.S. Compare to Other Countries?" Kaiser
Family Foundation, accessed July 1, 2018, https://www.kff.org/slideshow/
health-spending-in-the-u-s-as-compared-to-other-countries-slideshow/.

3. "How Does the Quality of the U.S. Healthcare System Compare to Other
Countries?" Bradley Sawyer and Selena Gonzalez, Health System Tracker,
May 22, 2017, https://www.healthsystemtracker.org/chart-collection/
quality-u-s-healthcare-system-compare-countries/?_sf_s=quality#item-start.

4. "'Big Government' Is Ever Growing, on the Sly," George Will, *National
Review*, February 25, 2017, https://www.nationalreview.com/2017/02/
federal-government-growth-continues-while-federal-employee-numbers-hold/.

5. "Ten Thousand Commandments 2017: An Annual Snapshot of the Federal
Regulatory State," Clyde Wayne Crews, Competitive Enterprise Institute, April
19, 2018, https://cei.org/10kc2018.

6. "Compilation of Patient Protection and Affordable Care Act," Health and Human
Services, June 9, 2018, https://www.hhs.gov/sites/default/files/ppacacon.pdf.

7. "How Many Pages of Regulations for 'Obamacare'?" Glenn Kessler, *Washington Post*, May 15, 2013, https://www.washingtonpost.com/blogs/fact-checker/post/how-many-pages-of-regulations-for-obamacare/2013/05/14/61eec914-bcf9-11e2-9b09-1638acc3942e_blog.html.

8. "Regulatory Overload Report," American Hospital Association, accessed June 20, 2018, https://www.aha.org/guidesreports/2017-11-03-regulatory-overload-report.

9. "World Health Statistics 2018: Monitoring Health for the SDGs," World Health Organization, accessed June 20, 2018, http://who.int/entity/gho/publications/world_health_statistics/2018/en/index.html.

10. "The World Fact Book," Central Intelligence Agency, accessed June 20, 2018, https://www.cia.gov/library/publications/the-world-factbook/fields/2075.html.

11. "Quick Facts," U.S. Census Bureau, accessed June 20, 2018, https://www.census.gov/quickfacts/fact/table/US/PST045217.

12. "Why Is the Opioid Epidemic Overwhelmingly White?" Noel King, host, NPR, November 4, 2017, https://www.npr.org/2017/11/04/562137082/why-is-the-opioid-epidemic-overwhelmingly-white.

13. "Hispanics' Health in the United States," Centers for Disease Control, accessed June 20, 2018, https://www.cdc.gov/media/releases/2015/p0505-hispanic-health.html.

14. "Treatment and Care for African Americans, American Diabetes Association, last updated October 1, 2014, http://www.diabetes.org/living-with-diabetes/treatment-and-care/high-risk-populations/treatment-african-americans.html.

15. "2017 Annual Report," America's Health Rankings, accessed July 1, 2018, https://www.americashealthrankings.org/learn/reports/2017-annual-report.

16. "Army Recruits from Southern States Most Unfit, Prone to Injury: Study," Richard Sisk, Military.com, January 16, 2018, https://www.military.com/daily-news/2018/01/16/army-recruits-southern-states-most-unfit-prone-injury-study.html.

17. "Medicare Program," U.S. Government Accountability Office, accessed July 1, 2018, https://www.gao.gov/highrisk/medicare_program/why_did_study.

18. "Addressing Improper Payments and the Tax Gap Would Improve the Government's Fiscal Position," U.S. Government Accountability Office, October 1, 2015, http://www.gao.gov/assets/680/672884.pdf.

19. "Medicare Fraud Strike Force," U.S. Department of Health and Human Services, accessed June 20, 2018, https://oig.hhs.gov/fraud/strike-force/.

20. "M&Ms," Mars, accessed June 20, 2018, http://www.mms.com/#product.

21. "Cheerios," General Mills, accessed June 20, 2018, http://www.cheerios.com/products.

22. "Top 20% of Americans Will Pay 87% of Income Tax," Laura Saunders, *The Wall Street Journal*, April 26, 2018, https://www.wsj.com/articles/top-20-of-americans-will-pay-87-of-income-tax-1523007001.

CHAPTER 7: VALUE-BASED CARE: AN ACADEMIC POLICY SOLUTION

1. "U.S. Health Care from a Global Perspective," David Squires, The Commonwealth Fund, October 8, 2015, http://www.commonwealthfund.org/publications/issue-briefs/2015/oct/us-health-care-from-a-global-perspective.

2. "Study Suggests High-Spending Doctors Could Do Less Without Harming Patients," Melanie Evans, *The Wall Street Journal*, March 13, 2017, https://www.wsj.com/articles/study-shows-high-spending-doctors-could-do-less-without-harming-patients-1489417200.

3. "House GOP Quietly Advances Key Elements of Tort Reform," Kimberly Kindy, *The Washington Post*, March 9, 2017, https://www.washingtonpost.com/national/house-gop-quietly-advances-key-elements-of-tort-reform/2017/03/09/d52213b2-0414-11e7-b1e9-a05d3c21f7cf_story.html.

4. "Bundled Payments for Care Improvement (BPCI) Initiative: General Information," Centers for Medicare & Medicaid Services, accessed June 20, 2018, https://innovation.cms.gov/initiatives/bundled-payments/.

5. "CMS Cancels Two Mandatory Pay Models and Scales Back a Third," Virgil Dickson, *Modern Healthcare*, August 15, 2017, http://www.modernhealthcare.com/article/20170815/news/170819935.

PART 2: AMERICA'S HEALTH CARE SYSTEM: THE DREAM PLAN

CHAPTER 8: LONGITUDINAL HEALTH CARE PLAN

1. "Surgery Center of Oklahoma," accessed June 21, 2018, https://surgerycenterok.com/.

CHAPTER 9: THE OBSOLESCENCE OF
TRADITIONAL HEALTH INSURANCE

1. "Shortage of Primary Care Physicians Could Threaten Patient Care," CBS News, August 2, 2017, https://www.cbsnews.com/news/ shortage-of-primary-care-physicians-could-threaten-patient-care/.

2. "Patient Engagement Survey: Improved Engagement Leads to Better Outcomes, but Better Tools Are Needed," Kevin G. Volpp, MD, PhD and Namita Seth Mohta, MD, NEJM Catalyst, May 12, 2016, http://catalyst.nejm.org/patient-engagement-report-improved-engagement-leads-better-outcomes-better-tools-needed/.

3. "Total Knee Replacement," Healthcare Bluebook, accessed June 21, 2018, https://healthcarebluebook.com/page_ProcedureDetails. aspx?cftid=31&g=Total%20Knee%20Replacement&directsearch=true.

4. "Skin Lesion Removal (malignant)," Healthcare Bluebook, June 21, 2018, https:// healthcarebluebook.com/page_ProcedureDetails.aspx?cftid=17&g=Skin%20 Lesion%20Removal%20(malignant)&directsearch=true.

5. "The Cost of HIV Treatment," Rachel Nall, Kimberly Holland, and Kristeen Cherney, Healthline, March 29, 2018, https://www.healthline.com/health/ hiv-aids/cost-of-treatment#1.

6. "HIV Cost-Effectiveness," Centers for Disease Control, accessed July 2, 2018, https://www.cdc.gov/hiv/programresources/guidance/costeffectiveness/ index.html.

7. "Type 2 Diabetes Can Be Cured Through Weight Loss, Newcastle University Finds," Sarah Knapton, *The Telegraph*, December 1, 2015, http://www.telegraph.co.uk/science/2016/03/14/ type-2-diabetes-can-be-cured-through-weight-loss-newcastle-unive/.

8. "Use of Physical and Intellectual Activities and Socialization in the Management of Cognitive Decline of Aging and in Dementia: A Review," Myuri Ruthirakuhan et al., *Journal of Aging Research* 2012 (2012): 384875, https:// www.ncbi.nlm.nih.gov/pmc/articles/PMC3549347/.

9. "The Effects of Grounding (Earthing) on Inflammation, the Immune Response, Wound Healing, and Prevention and Treatment of Chronic Inflammatory and Autoimmune Diseases," James L. Oschman, Gaétan Chevalier, and Richard Brown, *Journal of Inflammation Research* 8 (March 24, 2015), 83–96, https:// www.ncbi.nlm.nih.gov/pmc/articles/PMC4378297/.

10. "Chronic Disease Overview," Centers for Disease Control, accessed July 2, 2018, https://www.cdc.gov/chronicdisease/overview/index.htm.

11. "Charlie Gard: The Story of His Parents' Legal Fight," BBC News, July 27, 2017, https://www.bbc.com/news/health-40554462.

12. "Health/Patient and Family Support," Charity Navigator, accessed July 5, 2018, https://www.charitynavigator.org/index.cfm?bay=search. results&cgid=5&cuid=34.

CHAPTER 10: BUSINESS CASE FOR THE LHCP

1. "2017 Employer Health Benefits Survey," Kaiser Family Foundation, September 19, 2017, https://www.kff.org/report-section/ehbs-2017-summary-of-findings/.

2. "Despite Medicare, Seniors Will Pay More for Medical Care in Coming Years," Howard Gleckman, *Forbes*, March 30, 2017, https://www.forbes.com/sites/howardgleckman/2017/03/30/despite-medicare-seniors-will-pay-more-for-medical-care-in-coming-years/2/#4eadee4639ca.

3. "Questions and Answers for the Additional Medicare Tax," Internal Revenue Service, accessed July 2, 2018, https://www.irs.gov/businesses/small-businesses-self-employed/questions-and-answers-for-the-additional-medicare-tax.

4. "Questions and Answers on the Net Investment Income Tax," Internal Revenue Service, accessed July 2, 2018, https://www.irs.gov/newsroom/questions-and-answers-on-the-net-investment-income-tax.

5. "Commentary: The Case Against Employer-Sponsored Health Insurance," Janis Powers, myStatesman, May 23, 2018, https://www.mystatesman.com/news/opinion/commentary-the-case-against-employer-sponsored-health-insurance/DSyfBgvyTsx3YAcvY4LxKM/.

6. "Average Retirement Savings by Age," Daniel Kurt, RothIRA.com, accessed June 22, 2018, https://www.rothira.com/average-retirement-savings-age-2017.

CHAPTER 11: HOW THE DREAM PLAN CAN REDUCE COSTS IN HEALTH CARE

1. "2018 Alzheimer's Disease Facts and Figures," Alzheimer's Association*, accessed June 22, 2018, https://www.alz.org/facts/.

CHAPTER 12: PUBLIC HEALTH

1. "NHS Provokes Fury with Indefinite Surgery Ban for Smokers and Obese,"

Laura Donnelly, *The Telegraph*, October 17, 2017, http://www.telegraph.co.uk/news/2017/10/17/nhs-provokes-fury-indefinite-surgery-ban-smokers-obese/.

2. "Making Medicaid Recipients Work Being Pushed by Indiana, Other States," Maureen Groppe, *USA Today*, July 12, 2017, https://www.usatoday.com/story/news/politics/2017/07/12/making-medicaid-recipients-work-being-pushed-indiana-other-states/468326001/.

CHAPTER 13: MAKING OR BREAKING:
CRITICAL SUCCESS FACTORS

1. "Learning from CBO's History of Incorrect ObamaCare Projections," Brian Blase, *Forbes*, January 2, 2017, https://www.forbes.com/sites/theapothecary/2017/01/02/learning-from-cbos-history-of-incorrect-obamacare-projections/#1a761f2746a7.

2. "CFO's Fatal Flaw: Survey Finds 9 of 10 Hospital Executives Don't Know Their Cost," *Becker's Hospital Review*, accessed June 22, 2018, http://go.beckershospitalreview.com/cfos-fatal-flaw-survey-finds-9-of-10-hospital-executives-dont-know-their-cost.

3. "Can Declining Productivity Growth Be Reversed?" Bourree Lam, *The Atlantic*, March 14, 2017, https://www.theatlantic.com/business/archive/2017/03/productivity-interest-rate/519522/.LHCP Business Case Detail

LHCP BUSINESS CASE DETAIL

The data included in this section is the detail of the business case for the LHCP outlined in chapter 10. The chart outlines the dollars that a typical American and his or her employer pays into the health care system each year. Calculations related to per capita annual health care expenditures are also included. The Explanation of the Analysis provides line by line detail on the assumptions used to select these figures as well as the sources for the information.

Average income			
1	Average mean wage (gross pay)	$	50,620
2	Tax rate		25.00%
3	After-tax income	$	37,965

Categories of funding that could be directed to an LHCP					
		Percentage of contribution		Funds that could be contributed to an LHCP	
4		Low	High	Low	High
5	Personal budget				
6	Recommended after-tax income to budget for annual health care expenses	5.00%	10.00%	$ 1,898	$ 3,797
7	Component of recommended after-tax income budgeted for retirement savings that is typically used for health care expenses post-age 65	3.00%	4.00%	$ 1,139	$ 1,519
8	Subtotal, personal budget			$ 3,037	$ 5,315
9	Other sources				
10	Employee Medicare payroll tax (on gross pay)	1.45%	1.45%	$ 734	$ 734
11	Employer contribution to health insurance premiums			$ 5,486	$ 5,486
12	Subtotal, other sources			$ 6,220	$ 6,220
13	Total, personal budget and other sources			$ 9,257	$ 11,535
14	Average of categories of funds that could be directed to an LHCP			$	10,396

Estimation of health care expenditures per capita for 2017					
		Growth rate		Health care expenditures per capita	
15		Low	High	Low	High
16	Health care expenditures per capita, 2016			$	10,348
17	Estimate of health care expenditures per capita, 2017, using range of year over year growth rates from 2007 to 2016	2.21%	5.46%	$ 10,577	$ 10,913
18	Average of estimated low and high health care expenditures per capita, 2017			$	10,745

EXPLANATION OF ANALYSIS

1. Average mean wage is the gross pretax average annual income for all occupations in America as of May 2017 as reported by the Bureau of Labor Statistics. This figure is the average of about 142.5 million working Americans. "May 2017 National Occupational Employment and Wage Estimates United States," Bureau of Labor Statistics, accessed June 22, 2018, https://www.bls.gov/oes/current/oes_nat.htm.

2. Recommended household budgeting is based on after-tax income. Therefore, the average mean wage was adjusted by a typical tax rate. For an income around this level, estimates indicate a conservative tax rate of 25%.

3. After-tax income is the base income used for household budgeting.

4. Household budgeting percentages depend on a variety of factors, so I included a range of percentages of after-tax income and the associated dollar amounts for the analysis. Individuals may want to invest more or less, depending on their health status and based on the way they plan for their care as part of the design of their LHCP.

5. This first portion of the analysis identifies two categories in today's typical personal household budget that would be redirected to an LHCP.

6. Right now, experts indicate that individuals should budget somewhere between 5% to 10% of their after-tax income for personal health care expenses. All this money would be directed to an LHCP. Today, the cost that an individual would pay for monthly premiums would be funded from these dollars. The calculation in the chart makes sense because the individual contribution toward the average annual premium payment is $1,204. The figures on the previous page estimate that a person might budget between $1,898 to $3,797 for annual personal health care expenses. These figures should cover the cost of the premium, as well as other out-of-pocket expenses.

7. It is recommended that individuals invest between 15% to 20% of their income on savings. One of the most significant categories

of spending in retirement is health care, with some individuals spending 20% of their income on this category. I assumed 20% of the 15% to 20% in suggested savings would be directed into the LHCP. That equates to 3% to 4% of after-tax income.

8. This line sums the previous two figures.

9. Other sources capture either taxes paid by the individual or employer contributions to health care premiums.

10. This is the Medicare payroll tax that any employee must pay to the federal government, which is 1.45% of the average mean wage (not the after-tax income that the earlier savings estimates are based on).

11. This figure is the average annual employer contribution to health insurance premiums. It is a significant figure, and it may vary widely based on the employer. This is the largest contribution in the analysis. It's also the payment that has the least chance of being directly allocated to an individual for them to invest on their own. This issue is discussed at length in chapter 10.

12. This is the summation of the dollars associated with the Medicare payroll tax and the employer-sponsored premium contribution.

13. This line item sums up the two subcategories—dollars allocated to health care in a personal budget and contributions from other sources.

14. The average of the range of dollars identified in line 13 that could be directed to an LHCP is $10,396.

15. The data for the LHCP portion of the analysis is from 2017. The health care expenditures per capita figures from chapter 2, Chart 4, are from 2016. This section of the analysis estimates what the health care expenditures per capita costs might be for 2017.

16. Health care expenditures per capita in 2016 were $10,348.

17. Between 2007 and 2016, the year-over-year increase in health care expenditures per capita ranged from 2.12% to 5.46%. Health care expenditures per capita were estimated for 2017 based on the

range of potential annual increases applied to the 2016 base figure of $10,348.

18. This shows the average of the range of estimated health care expenditures per capita calculations for 2017.

ABOUT THE AUTHOR

Janis Powers graduated from Yale and earned masters' degrees in business and architecture from the University of Michigan. She grew up in New York and has lived the majority of her adult life in Texas. She will listen to anyone's side of a story.

Her first book, *Mama's Got a Brand New Job*, is a novel about one woman's transition from power professional to power mom. It's based on a true story.

Janis is often spotted running around her neighborhood in Austin. She's an avid cook who's obsessed with current affairs and planning trips to faraway places. Her two children are two of her best friends.